Meeting the Needs of Children with Disabilities

D0221616

Children with disabilities have needs that reflect the needs of every child of their age or stage of development, but in addition they will have other needs that are unique and special to them. This text provides the reader with an insight into the needs of children with both physical and learning disabilities, particularly within an acute care setting.

The book considers the principles that underpin the fundamental aspects of care delivery to children with special needs, and areas of knowledge and practical skill covered include:

- Social and historical context
- Challenging assumptions
- Best practice for giving news to parents
- Communication methods
- Play and movement
- Nutrition and feeding
- Boundary setting
- Respite care
- Transitions into adult services

Meeting the Needs of Children with Disabilities covers practice areas identified by the English National Board as essential for student nurses. It will also be invaluable for qualified nurses, other health professionals working with children with disabilities and for those who work in respite care settings and residential schools.

Helen K. Warner is an Early Intervention Nurse for Services for Children and Young People with Learning Disabilities and Challenging Behaviour and Their Families, in East Kent. She trained at the Hospital for Sick Children, Great Ormond Street, London and has worked as a Senior Staff Nurse in both Acute Paediatrics and Child Development.

Meeting the Needs of Children with Disabilities

Families and professionals facing the challenge together

Edited by
Helen K. Warner

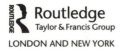

Routledge
Taylor & Francis Group

LONDON AND NEW YORK

For my dear friend, Kathy

First published 2006
by Routledge
2 Park Square, Milton Park, Abingdon, Oxon OX14 4RN

Simultaneously published in the USA and Canada
by Routledge
270 Madison Ave, New York, NY 10016

Routledge is an imprint of the Taylor & Francis Group

© 2006 Helen K. Warner selection and editorial matter;
individual chapters the contributors

Typeset in Goudy by RefineCatch Ltd, Bungay, Suffolk
Printed and bound in Great Britain by
TJ International Ltd, Padstow, Cornwall

British Library Cataloguing in Publication Data
A catalogue record for this book is available from the British Library

Library of Congress Cataloging in Publication Data
A catalog record has been requested for this book

ISBN10: 0–415–28037–0 (hbk)
ISBN10: 0–415–28038–9 (pbk)

ISBN13: 9–78–0–415–28037–2 (hbk)
ISBN13: 9–78–0–415–28038–9 (pbk)

Contents

List of tables and figures

Tables

Figures

Contributors

Helen K. Warner trained at the Hospital for Sick Children, Great Ormond Street, London. After qualifying she married and raised a family prior to returning to nursing in 1979, as Staff Nurse and subsequently Senior Staff Nurse, on the Paediatric Unit in East Kent, until 1997. During that time Helen returned to college to update her skills, also developing a growing interest in children with disabilities. From 1997–2002 she managed an Early Intervention Unit for children aged 0–3 years, within a Child Development Centre, during which time she completed a University of Kent Certificate in Counselling Studies Course. Helen has had three articles published and won an East Kent Hospitals NHS Trusts 3rd prize for innovations in working practice in October 2000. Helen's team was also highly commended in the 2001 Trust Awards. Helen has presented two papers at the RCN Paediatric Conferences. She has been in her current role as Early Intervention Nurse, Services for Children and Young People with Learning Disabilities and Challenging Behaviour and Their Families, in East Kent, since November 2002.

Catherine Bernal is a Registered Nurse for Learning Disability, currently employed as Senior Lecturer in Learning Disability by Canterbury Christ Church University College. She completed her pre-registration studies in 1985, and (allowing for five years spent studying unrelated subjects in higher education) has many years' experience of managing residential support, largely in the private sector. Her particular interests in practice are services for clients with profound and complex needs, including physical disabilities and challenging behaviour.

Catherine has been in her current post since April 2000, and has developed a research interest in the education of aspirant mental health, child and adult nurses with regard to supporting people with learning disabilities.

Catherine has had three articles published and a fourth is in press.

Kim Broster was a practising Specialist Health Visitor for children with special needs, working for Maidstone and Weald NHS Primary Care Trust, at the time of writing. This post included supporting parents following diagnosis of their child's special needs, including giving relevant information and introducing services, and acting as a resource for pre-school-age children with complex special needs and their families. She worked in consultation with other health professionals to coordinate care plans, including inter-agency planning and chairing of planning meetings. She was involved in training and raising awareness regarding issues related to disability for professional and voluntary groups, for example the emotional impact of disability on a family and the Key Worker Role. She facilitated a support group for parents and is responsible for the organising and co-ordinating of the referrals meeting and was a core team member of a multi-disciplinary feeding clinic.

In this post she facilitated a service user group for parents of children with special needs receiving frequent in-patient hospital services. The work with this parent group included the development for ward staff of a detailed care plan for children with complex needs, which was presented at the RCN Society of Paediatric Nursing Conference, September 2000, Bristol, as 'Working in Partnership: collaborating in the development of parent held documentation that facilitates the nursing of children with special needs.' She is also Lead Nurse in Maidstone and Weald NHS Primary Care Trust for this area of pre-school children with special needs and supervisor for group child protection supervision.

Kim currently works for Gravesham SureStart.

Claire Thurgate: following qualification, Claire gained experience within acute paediatrics, staffing on children's wards in East Kent, before moving into caring for the child with disabilities and complex needs. During her work with children with complex needs Claire was instrumental in the development of a health funded respite service. Claire now has a lecturer's post in Child Health Nursing at Canterbury Christ Church University College, where she aims to raise awareness amongst paediatric nurses of caring for children with disabilities.

Claire has presented two papers regarding respite care at RCN Paediatric Conferences and has had two papers about respite care accepted for publication.

Acknowledgements

First of all I would like to acknowledge the children and families who have been the inspiration for this book. We are immensely grateful to them for sharing their stories with us, particularly when they have often had to work through personal trauma and emotional pain in order to do so. As professionals it is a privilege to share their stories, which serves to enhance our professional work.

Grateful thanks to Kay Hutchfield without whom this book would never have got started.

Thanks also to everyone at Routledge with whom I came into contact, for all their help and understanding.

I am grateful to the Physiotherapists, Occupational therapists and the Speech and Language therapists from the Mary Sheridan Centre, Canterbury, for their advice, support, and critical reading of relevant chapters, in particular Katrina Rogers, Gilly Martin and Anne Kirby.

Thanks also to my colleagues in the Services for Children and Young People with Learning Disabilities and Challenging Behaviour and Their Families Team who have taught me so much. Their influence has also been inspirational, with a special thank you to Gunnar Sivertson, Psychologist, for his painstaking help and advice.

Last but not least, a special thank you to Dave, for his patience, tea and sympathy.

Helen K. Warner

Introduction

The origins of this book lie with the parents of a Regular Users of Paediatric Services group, who wanted to improve health professionals' understanding of their children who had 'special' or 'additional needs'. Their participation has resulted in a significant improvement in the information available to nurses caring for their children in the local general children's ward. This book aims to share some of the lessons that have been learnt through the work of this group.

In addition, lessons learned by clinicians working in the community and within a Child Development Centre are also shared. It is only by listening to parents and taking note of their concerns that professionals can begin to understand the needs of children with disabilities and their families.

This book is concerned with professionals and families sharing their expertise to provide the reader with an insight into the needs of children with both physical and learning disabilities within the context of the acute hospital setting. The book also aims to provide the reader with an understanding that the acute setting may only play a relatively small part in the lives of some children whose care, nevertheless, may require the input of many professionals from different disciplines and agencies in the community. For some of these children a reason for their disability may have been identified e.g. Downs syndrome or autism. However, for many, the cause of their disability may not be known, and this fact may affect their parents' ability in coming to terms with the reality of their child's care.

For a few children the nature of their disability may be so severe that it affects their ability to live an independent life, such as severe cerebral palsy or a genetic condition such as Batten's disease. The number of children with such severe disability is not large, but they are lifelong users of children's in-patient and out-patient services, and, as such, require special consideration. They have needs that reflect the needs of every child of their age or stage of development, but in addition they will have other needs that are unique and special to them. In the acute care context the families are usually the primary source of expert information in regard to the child's daily care, but it is important to remember that the parents are also in need of care and support when their child is acutely ill.

This book will consider the principles that underpin the fundamental aspects of care delivery to children with special needs, in the acute care setting. These will include those areas identified by the English National Board (ENB 2000) as necessary areas of knowledge and skills needed by student nurses, and, it could be argued, by qualified nurses and other health professionals too, who care for children with learning difficulties.

Before moving on it would seem appropriate to begin where this book began, with individual children. Only by understanding the perspective of the child and family can we, as health professionals, begin to provide the care that these children and their families deserve.

The following chapters will focus on the practicalities as well as the theories of caring/nursing children with disabilities. There is a chapter on the social and historical context with the focus on the continually changing attitudes towards the disabled as the social model of disability is more readily adopted. Following on from this, Chapter 3 challenges the assumption that having a child with disabilities is necessarily a tragedy and Chapter 4 discusses the ethics relating to the allocation of resources for children with disabilities. Chapter 5 discusses best practice for giving the initial diagnosis to the family as recommended in *Right From The Start* (Leonard 1994). Building a trusting relationship is a prerequisite for working with children and families, and the next chapter will focus on how trust can be helped to develop. Play is central to the development of children (Roberts 1995) and if the opportunity to play is restricted or denied, children can suffer developmentally (The Children's Play Council 1998). Thus another chapter will discuss the increased importance of play for children with disabilities when in hospital, and also how children learn to move and to play. Other chapters will consider some of the problems disabled children may have in obtaining sufficient nutrition to sustain growth and make some practical suggestions for helping children to eat and drink. Following on from this there will be a discussion of communication methods in order to dispel the myth that if a child does not speak, he/she cannot communicate. Further chapters will focus on attachment and boundary setting; the assessment of pain; managing difficult behaviour in the acute setting; the importance of respite care; the transition into adult services; and finally, the way forward for services as they strive to work more closely together.

Where there is little scientific evidence, justification for practice may come from consensus among appropriate experts (Hemihelp 1999) since this consensus may be in advance of published research, due to the time delay in the publication process. It has been suggested that intuition may also be important (Harries and Harries 2001); the knowledge and experience of experts enabling them to make judgements based on apparently little evidence but using the often forgotten factor of common sense (Hemihelp 1999).

References

English National Board (2000) *Education in Focus: Strengthening pre-registration nursing and midwifery education*, London: ENB.

Harries, P. A. and Harries, C. (2001) 'Studying Clinical Reasoning, Part 2: Applying Social Judgement Theory', *British Journal Occupational Therapy* June 64. 6: 285–292.

Hemihelp (1999) *Recommendations for Minimum Standards of Healthcare in Children with Cerebral Palsy*, Surrey: Bell Pottinger Healthcare.

Leonard, A. (1994) *Right from the Start*, London: Scope.

Roberts, P. (1995) 'Goofing Off', *Psychology Today*, July/Aug, 34–41.

The Children's Play Council (1998) *The New Charter for Children's Play*: London: The Children's Society.

1 Meeting the fundamental needs of children with disabilities

Helen K. Warner

Raising awareness

Attitudes towards disability within British society are changing from those that were disempowering and excluding, to a more enlightened approach based on the social model of disability. This chapter will explore the recent changes within the contexts of acute hospital care and a child assessment centre.

Current attitudes towards disability appear different from those existing in the 1960s that hid away the physically and learning-disabled in large institutions, and labelled them as the 'socially dead' (BBC2 1999). However, preconceived ideas and prejudices surrounding disability still exist and are difficult to change. This can create problems for parents striving to obtain the best services for their children with disabilities.

Working within a Child Assessment Centre, the writer became very aware that families often still have to fight to get what they want for their children regardless of whether it is a medical, educational or social service to which they are entitled. Parents need to quickly learn to be assertive, and to find the energy to challenge a system and resources that do not always meet their requirements. All this in addition to caring for a child with special/additional needs may leave the parents feeling mentally and physically exhausted.

Giddens (1995) stated that: 'in a society that places high value on youth, vitality and physical attractiveness, non-participants become invisible' (p. 651). This raises the question of how the 'invisible' are made more visible (Warner 2000). The establishment of a Disability Advisory Group (DAG) in 1998 for every NHS Trust could be seen as one way of pushing disability up the social and political agenda, but it gained little more than a passing mention from the media. The formation of the Disability Rights Commission (DRC) in April 2000, by the Department of Employment and Education, appeared to suffer a similar fate.

The DRC was established to ensure that the Disability Discrimination Act (DDA, DoH 1995) was revised and discrimination eliminated. It also had the power to investigate any allegations of discrimination. It was a crucial step in the struggle for the disabled to be given civil rights and yet attracted little media interest.

In contrast, a great deal of media coverage was given to remarks made by the footballer, Glen Hoddle (*The Times*, editorial, 1 February 1999). Hoddle suggested that disabled people are being punished for sins in a former life, which must have caused great offence. The Prime Minister became involved and Hoddle lost his job as Manager of the England Football Team. However, the profile on disability issues was only briefly raised.

Raising awareness of disability issues is a continuing process and one which still has a long way to go. Disabled people remain disadvantaged in many areas of life as the facts from the Department of Social Security (DSS 1999) shown in Table 1.1 below illustrate.

Education

Education is another area where the disabled child may be disadvantaged. Following publication of the *Within Reach 1* study (1992) and *Within Reach 2* survey (1993) carried out for the National Union of Teachers (NUT) and the Scope Advisory and Assessment Service for People with Cerebral Palsy, a third study, *Within Reach 3* (2001) was commissioned. This revealed a lack of knowledge about the accessibility of schools, even though the Education Act (1981) had set out to make appropriate provision in mainstream schools, wherever possible, for children with special educational needs (Lennard 1992).

This provision was to be based on individual assessment of children's needs, with parents sharing in the assessment, planning and decision-making process. However, the reality is that procedures for assessment and statementing are so complex that there is a real risk of delay in reaching a conclusion. Even when a decision is reached, the Scope study found that there was often disparity between parents' and professionals' views, and parents feeling distressed to find themselves in conflict with the agencies ostensibly set up to help them (Lennard 1992).

Many local education authorities (LEAs) were found to have been making decisions about children's education on the basis of the resources they had at their disposal. Segregated education is a cheaper option, regardless of the

Table 1.1 Disadvantages faced by disabled people

- Only 18 per cent of primary schools and 8% of secondary schools have complete wheelchair access.
- Nearly half (47 per cent) of essential equipment needed to help some disabled people communicate is not funded by statutory organisations.
- Over 50 per cent of disabled people have difficulty using public transport.
- Households with a disabled person have an income 20–30 per cent lower than that of the average household.
- Disabled people are seven times more likely to be out of work.
- One in three disabled people have been refused access to a public place e.g. pub, restaurant, theatre or leisure centre.

child's need to be integrated into society. In addition, teachers in mainstream schools were found to be inadequately prepared to integrate disabled children into their classes.

Inclusive education is a prerequisite for establishing an inclusive society. The change towards an education system designed to include everyone rather than making disabled children 'fit' into a system not designed with their needs in mind has, at last, the support of government, with the introduction of a policy for increased inclusion of children with disabilities into mainstream schools (Gibson and McGahren 2001).

The Schools Access Initiative (SAI) launched in 1995 by the government to provide funding to improve access to the premises of mainstream schools has been welcomed. However, education is not just about access, but is a process which enables disabled children to receive their rights and entitlements and to feel a sense of achievement which will increase their self-esteem and self-confidence. To provide this, teachers and others involved in school education need to be trained in disability awareness. Extra help and support is needed to enable children with special educational needs (SEN) to get the most out of the educational system alongside their peers, but they often only get the support they need through enforceable statements of SEN. However, the recent changes in education have been made with the aim of extra support to schools so that the statementing process is fast becoming obsolete even though there will always be some children whose needs will not be adequately met within the mainstream environment. There is also an increasing emphasis on academic instruction in early childhood education that is based on misconceptions about early learning (Elkind 1986; 1987). Bredekamp (1987) asserts that this is incompatible with a curriculum that is based on developmentally appropriate practice within child-centred programmes. This is discussed further by David, Moir and Herbert (1997) together with the implications for higher levels of staff who are well trained and well paid. However, the fear remains that sufficient support is still not in place and a generation of children will have been set up to fail.

This situation appears to reflect what happened when the large mental institutions were closed down in the 1970s and 1980s and the inmates moved into a society that was as ill prepared to receive them into their midst, as they themselves were to find themselves suddenly leaving what had been their only home for most of their lives.

However the government's strategy for SEN, *Removing Barriers to Achievement* (DfES 2004) aims, as promised in the Green Paper, *Every Child Matters* (DfES 2003), to realise the vision of a society where all children have the opportunity to achieve their full potential through good quality childcare, early education and school. The strategy aims to personalise learning for children with SEN by making education more innovative and responsive to their diverse needs. It covers all aspects of school life, and incorporates actions that Sure Start will be taking to improve access to childcare and leisure facilities for children aged 0–16 years who have disabilities. The main features of the strategy regarding childcare and education include action on:

- Improving information for parents and childcare/early education providers.
- Collecting and disseminating good practice through work with Children's Trusts, Connexions and local authorities (Connexions is an advice and guidance service for all 13–19 year olds).
- Helping families meet additional costs.
- Improving access to training for the childcare workforce.

The NHS

NHS Hospital Trusts, as a result of the DDA (1995) and the DRC, should now include disability awareness training for all new staff in addition to taking measures to raise the awareness of their existing staff. Trusts need to work in partnership with local disability groups to ensure that any obstacles in the environment are removed, so that access to services is no more difficult for the disabled than it is for any other service user. This includes signs at wheelchair level, lift controls at an appropriate height for users, information leaflets / notices in contrasting colours and large print, with loop systems for the hearing impaired, and the availability of interpreters as necessary. In short, to show disabled people the respect they have a right to expect and to allow them to maintain the degree of independence they have. This also applies to the children with disabilities who find themselves in the acute healthcare setting.

Acute in-patient services

It was estimated that there were approximately 360,000 children with disabilities and that 159,000 of these had multiple impairments (Office of Public and Census Surveys 1989). These children are three times more likely to require a hospital admission than their peers, with a predicted stay of seven rather than two days (Hirst and Baldwin 1994). The number of these children is also increasing with the technological advances in medical and nursing care (Hancock 1995; Kirk 1999; Olsen and Maslin-Prothero 2001).

Interestingly, in the year 2000 the NHS Executive were unable to provide any figures for hospital admissions of children with physical and/or learning disabilities or any indication of their length of stay (Kingdom and Mayfield 2001), and yet these children will be lifelong users of the health and social services. However the Department of Health (2000) estimated that there were 549,800 children under the age of 19 years with special needs. Thus, although in the past student nurses may not have come across many of these children in the acute hospital setting, this is unlikely to remain the case. This view is supported by research that demonstrates that a dis-proportionate number of children with disabilities are very young (Roberts and Lawton 2001), and up to 50 per cent of severely disabled children under 2 years old are dependent on at least one piece of medical equipment (Beresford 1995).

However, Nessa (2004) concluded that good quality and accurate data is unavailable at a national level so that long-term trends in children and young people with disabilities have not been established. It has therefore not been possible to accurately assess standards in the development and delivery of services generally and in particular in meeting the needs of families with technologically dependent children.

Villarneal and Johnson (1995) state that it is a challenge to provide quality care for the physically and/or learning-disabled child, whether acutely ill or requiring elective surgery. Hewson (1997) argues that, although students may have been academically prepared to understand the medical implications, they may not know how to nurse these children, or how to support their parents (Swallow and Jacoby 2001). This book aims to try to bridge that knowledge gap.

The risks of hospital admission

The risk of emotional harm to young children when admitted to hospital has been recognised and well documented, owing much to the work of Bowlby (1971) and Robertson (1970). In spite of numerous reports and government guidelines dating from the Platt Report (1959) to the present day (Table 1.2), there are still some areas that are failing to address the special needs of children and their families (Glasper and Powell 1996).

As Professor Kennedy's Report (2001) stated, children's services remain a 'Cinderella' service after 25 years, and children have died as a result of a combination of 'general failings in the NHS' as well as 'individual failing'. However, if Kennedy's (2001) recommendations are met in full, it will demonstrate that what has been learned from the deaths of those children in Bristol has been acted upon in order to prevent any other deaths resulting from inadequate resources and insufficient numbers of staff being trained in the care of children. Although Kennedy was referring to children generally and not specifically to children and young people with disabilities, it is clear that inadequate resources and numbers of appropriately trained staff will have an impact on the care of these most vulnerable children, both in the acute setting and in the community.

Children with disabilities are children first and foremost, having all the needs of any other child. However, for the child with disabilities, all of those difficulties faced by any other child in hospital may be hugely magnified. As well as the psychological regression, which may affect any hospitalised child, the child with disability may also experience physical regression and loss of independence due to poor positioning and a lack of appropriate stimulation.

Table 1.2 Government guidelines/reports: 1959–2001

Platt, H. (1959)	*The Welfare of Children in Hospital*, Report of the Committee on Child Health Services, London, HMSO.
DOH (1976)	*Fit for the Future*, Report of the Court Committee on Child Health Services, London, HMSO.
National Association for the Welfare of Children in Hospital (1984)	*Charter for Children in Hospital*, London, NAWCH.
DOH (1991a)	*Welfare of children and young people in hospital*, London, HMSO.
DOH (1991b)	*The Children Act 1989: An Introductory Guide for the NHS*, London, HMSO.
Action for Sick Children (1992)	*Ten Targets for the 1990's*, London, ASC.
Audit Commission (1993)	*Children First: A study of hospital services for local authorities and the NHS*, London, HMSO.
Clothier, Sir C. (1994)	*Inquiry relating to deaths and injuries on the children's ward at Grantham and Kesteven General Hospital*, London, HMSO.
Royal College of Nursing (1994)	*The care of sick children: A review of the Guidelines in the wake of the Allitt Inquiry*, London, HMSO.
Rcn (1995)	*Paediatric Nursing: A Philosophy of Care*, London, Rcn.
DOH (1996)	*The Patients Charter, Services for Children and Young People*. London, HMSO.
House Of Commons Select Committee (1966/7)	*Hospital services for children and young people*, vol. 1, London, HMSO.
DOH (1997)	*The New NHS: Modern and Dependable*, London, HMSO.
DOH (1998)	*A First Class Service: Quality in the NHS*, London, HMSO.
DOH (1999)	*Making a Difference*, London, HMSO.
United Kingdom Central Council for Nursing, Midwifery and Health Visiting (1999)	*Fit for Practice*, London, UKCC.
DOH (2001)	*Valuing People: A new strategy for learning disability for the 21st century*, London, HMSO.
Kennedy, Prof. I. (2001)	*Learning from Bristol: Report of the Public Inquiry into Children's Heart Surgery at the Bristol Royal Infirmary 1984–1995*, London, HMSO.

Poor positioning can lead to increased spasticity, which in turn may lead to increased disability, impair respiration and digestion and result in poor dietary intake and therefore also nutritional status. Poor positioning can also limit the child's ability to communicate and reduce the opportunity to play, resulting in negative self-esteem. Chest and urinary infections and indeed simply feeling unwell and/or constipated can also increase spasticity. There is also the potential problem of pressure sores developing, which will cause added pain and distress to the child.

Impact on parents

For parents, the uncertainty generated by the unpredictability of their child's future quality of life may impede their psychological management of the condition (Cohen 1997). It may also initiate a grief response in mothers (Gibson 1995), which may be repeatedly triggered with every hospital admission. Repetitive questions from medical and nursing staff may serve to exacerbate any feelings of grief and anger (Rees 1998). In addition, Coyne (1995) found that parents' self-confidence and coping ability were undermined by scepticism from professionals, non-negotiation of roles and inadequate provision of information. An important finding of Gibson (1995) was how isolated mothers often are and this also may be exacerbated with a hospital admission if parents are allowed to continue to carry the burden of care, and possibly feel unable to take a break, even when they are offered the opportunity to do so. It is important to remember that the child's family is also in need of care, and especially when their child is in hospital. Dale (1996) advocates a negotiated partnership model that stresses the importance of a whole-family approach; an approach which has to take into account changing family dynamics.

Minimising the risks

Professionals need to be sensitive, choose their words with care and not make any assumptions about the child or his/her family. As one parent has said, the most supportive people are those who have come alongside and are willing to listen, and yet do not hold back out of fear for saying the wrong thing (Kingdom and Mayfield 2001).

The aim of the following chapters is to enable children's nurses and other health professionals to minimise the risks of a hospital admission for the child with severe disability, and to maintain his/her existing independence/ skills as far as possible. An outline of the areas to consider when assessing the needs of a child with complex disabilities will be provided along with the type of questions that may need to be asked in order to obtain the information needed to effectively care for the child.

No one discipline can meet the needs of children with disabilities in isolation. Ward staff must be aware that there may already be many professionals/agencies involved in individual children's care and that it is vital to keep the communication channels open between them. It is also essential to remember and acknowledge that parents are experts in their child's care and may have much to teach nurses and other healthcare professionals about their child's daily care needs. With this acknowledgement it is possible to treat parents as equal partners in the care of their child.

Nurses who demonstrate respect for the experience, abilities and strengths of parents and a willingness to actively listen and hear what parents have to say can help to develop a satisfying relationship with them (Darbyshire 1994).

In the same way, acknowledging and valuing the input of those other professionals involved will enable good relationships to develop throughout the multi-disciplinary team. Nurses are in a good position to facilitate this by being willing and able to discuss with parents and explain all that is proposed, planned and agreed by the team in a sensitive and non-patronising way that is easy to understand (Darbyshire 1994). It is vital for nurses to understand that different disciplines, and also different agencies, overlap in their knowledge and expertise, each having a small piece of the whole picture, so that it is only when there is a coming together of the different perspectives, including the child and family's perspective, that the child can be viewed as a whole and cared for holistically.

References

BBC2 (1999) *The Disabled Century*, Television Documentary.

Beresford, B. (1995) *Expert Opinions: a national survey of parents caring for a severely disabled child*, Bristol: The Policy Press.

Bowlby, J. (1971) *Attachment and Loss* (Vol. 1) Harmondsworth: Penguin.

Bredekamp, S. (1987) *Developmentally Appropriate Practice in Early Childhood Programmes Serving Children from Birth through Age Eight*, National Association for the Education of Young Children: Washington DC.

Casey, A. (2001) 'Six words say it all' *Paediatric Nursing*, 13(7) 3.

Cohen, M. H. (1997) 'The stages of pre-diagnostic period in chronic life threatening childhood illness: a process analysis', *Research in Nursing and Health* 18: 39–48.

Coyne, I. T. (1995) 'Partnership in care: parents' views of participation in their hospitalised child's care', *Journal of Clinical Nursing* 4: 71–79.

Dale, N. (1996) *Working with Families of Children with Special Needs: Partnership and Practice*, London: Routledge.

Darbyshire, P. (1994) *Living with a sick child in hospital*, London: Chapman and Hall.

David, T., Moir, J., Herbert, E., (1997) 'Curriculum issues in early childhood: implications for families', in B. Carpenter (ed.) *Families in Context*, London: David Fulton.

Department for Education and Skills (2003) *Every Child Matters*, Nottingham: DFES.

Department for Education and Skills (2004) *Removing Barriers to Achievement – the Government's strategy for SEN*, Nottingham, DFES.

Department of Health (1991) *The Children Act 1989: An Introductory Guide for the NHS*, London: HMSO.

Department of Health (1995) *Disability Discrimination Act*, London: HMSO.

Department of Health (2000) *Quality Protects: Disabled Children, Numbers and Categories*, London: HMSO.

Department of Social Security (1999) *Disability in Great Britain*, London: DSS.

Elkind, D. (1986) 'Formal education and early childhood education: an essential difference', *Phi Delta Kappan* 67: 631–6.

Elkind, D. (1987) *Miseducation: Preschoolers at Risk*, Boston: Allyn and Bacon.

Gibson, C. H. (1995) 'The process of empowerment in mothers of chronically ill Children', *Journal of Advanced Nursing*, 21: 1201–1210.

Gibson, C. and McGahren, Y. (2001) *When your Child has Special Needs: A Guide for Parents who Care for a Child with a Disability, Special Need or Rare Disorder*, London: Contact a Family.

Giddens, A. (1995) *Sociology* (2nd edn), Oxford: Polity Press.

Glasper, E. and Powell, C. (1996) 'The Challenge of The Children's Charter: rhetoric vs reality', *British Journal of Nursing* 5(1) 26–29.

Hancock, J. (1995) 'Prematurity: Long term effects', *Paediatric Nursing* 7: 10, 14.

Hewson, D. (1997) *Children's Nurses: perceptions of their preparation for the care of children with disabilities*, Dept. Nursing Studies, University of Nottingham.

Hirst, M. and Baldwin, S. (1994) *Unequal Opportunities: Growing up Disabled*, The Social Policy Research Group, London: HMSO.

Kennedy, I. (2001) *Learning from Bristol: Report of the Public Inquiry into Children's Heart Surgery at the Bristol Royal Infirmary 1984–1995*, London: HMSO.

Kingdom, S. and Mayfield, C. (2001) 'Complex Disabilities: Parents Preparing Professionals', *Paediatric Nursing* 13(7) Sept. 34–38.

Kirk, S. (1999) 'Caring for Children with Specialised Healthcare Needs in the Community: The Challenges for Primary Care', *Health and Social Care in the Community* 7(5) 350–357.

Lennard, A. (1992) *A Hard Act to Follow*, The Spastics Society for People with Cerebral Palsy.

National Union of Teachers/Scope (1992) *Within Reach 1: Access for disabled children to mainstream schools*, Joint Report by SCOPE and NUT.

National Union of Teachers/Scope (1993) *Within Reach 2: The School Survey*, Joint Report by SCOPE and NUT.

National Union of Teachers/Scope, PricewaterhouseCoopers, Dept. of Education and Employment (2001) *Within Reach 3: An Evaluation of the Schools Access Initiative* London: NUT.

Nessa N. (2004) 'Disability', chapter 10 in *The Health of Children and Young People*, Office for National Statistics (March).

Office of Public and Census Surveys (1989) *Report 3: Prevalence of Disability*, OPCS.

Olsen, R. and Maslin-Prothero, P. (2001) 'Dilemmas in the provision of own home respite support for parents of young children with complex healthcare needs: Evidence from evaluation', *Journal of Advanced Nursing* 34(5) 603–610.

Rees, S. (1998) 'A Parent's Experience of Hospital Admission', Royal College of Nursing Children with Disabilities Special Interest Group Annual Conference, Dec. 12.

Roberts, K. and Lawton, D. (2001) 'Acknowledging the extra care parents give their disabled children', *Childcare, Health and Development* 27(4), 307–319.

Robertson, J. (1970) *Young Children in Hospital* (2nd edn), London: Tavistock.

Spastics Society (1994) *Right from the start*, London: The Spastics Society.

Swallow, V. and Jacoby, A. (2001) 'Mothers' coping in chronic childhood illness; The effects of pre-symptomatic diagnosis of vesico-ureteric reflux', *Journal of Advanced Nursing* 33(1) 69–78.

The Times (1999) 'Hoddle Must Go', (editorial, 1 February), Times Newspapers Ltd.

Villarneal, P. and Johnson, C. P. (1995) 'Nursing care of children with developmental disabilities having surgery', *Seminars in Peri-Operative Nursing* 4(2) 96–111.

Warner, H. (2000) 'Making the Invisible, Visible', *Journal of Child Health Care* 4(3) 123–126.

2 The sociological and historical context of disability

Catherine Bernal

What is disability?

The Disability Discrimination Act (DoH 1995) proclaims 'see the person' rather than the disability, and there is no doubt that in Britain there is a culture that largely supports a social model of disability that places more importance on the individual than on their diagnosis, impairment or disability. This model has been 'hard won' by the advocates of disability rights, and this chapter will consider the means by which it was achieved. It is also the intention to communicate to the reader a clear picture of the children to whom this book refers, and to propose a user-friendly definition of the term disability.

Defining disability

It seems reasonable to assume that any attempt to define disability will be value-laden, and will reflect the context within which it has been developed. Consider the following definitions:

> Any restriction or lack (resulting from an impairment) of ability to perform an activity in the manner or within the range considered normal for a human being
>
> (WHO 1980)

> a child is disabled if 'he is blind, deaf or dumb, suffers from mental disorder of any kind or is substantially and permanently handicapped by illness, injury or congenital deformity or such other disability as may be prescribed'
>
> (*Children Act*, DoH 1989: 52)

> impairment that substantially limits one or more of the major life activities
>
> (Americans with Disabilities Act 1990, quoted in Barnes *et al.* 1999)

Such definitions may seem sensible, but are focused on assumptions of biophysiological standards of normality. They imply that it is the individual's impairment rather than society's attitude or willingness to accept diversity that inhibits his or her ability to overcome some of the challenges disability presents. These definitions could be said to reflect the *medical* model of disability.

The *social* model of disability moves away from defining a disabled person by his or her inherent deficiencies, and proposes that it is society that disables people by its lack of provision for their needs, negative assumptions and the erection of 'disabling barriers' (Swain *et al.* 1997). A disabled sociologist has claimed, that 'disability is socially produced' (Oliver 1992). This perspective is shared by others and has led to the development of an alternative definition of disability:

> The disadvantage or restriction of activity caused by a contemporary social organisation which takes little or no account of people who have physical impairments and thus excludes them from participation in the mainstream of social activities.
>
> (UPIAS 1976: 3–4)

This definition, proposed by the Union of the Physically Impaired Against Segregation, overturns conventional notions by suggesting that no individual is disabled except by the society in which he or she lives. Such an approach is reinforced by the enormously varied interpretations different world cultures place upon disabled members of their communities; in Martha's Vineyard, for example, the result of a high proportion of children born congenitally deaf was the acquisition by the whole community of sign language in addition to spoken English – not the segregation and disabling of those affected (Groce cited in Barnes *et al.* 1999: 16).

It is true that 'disability is not measles' (Rioux and Bach 1994), but from a practical standpoint it is necessary to find a word that identifies those people for whom the whole of society – including the healthcare professions – needs to make extraordinary provision in order to support their *enablement* needs. However, an exploration of the social model of disability does not help the reader of this book to identify the precise nature of the client group to which it refers. Suffice to say that for the writers of this book, the children to whose needs it is addressed are those with multiple impairments – be they mental or physical – that result in the disabling of the child in contemporary British society. We assume that these impairments are lifelong, or at least expected to be; and include those diagnosed as autistic (who are likely in addition to be learning disabled). However, we exclude children disabled solely by mental illness or any other condition generally considered treatable.

What has been offered is not, admittedly, a clean and tidy definition of 'disability'; as demonstrated, it is perhaps impossible to achieve this in a practical context. The writers hope, however, that what is presented in the following pages will assist the reader, possibly new to the field, in meeting the needs of children with multiple impairments and their families.

The historical context: from changelings to agents of change

T. S. Eliot, writing shortly before the outbreak of the Second World War, clearly felt that an exploration of the past was essential to the understanding of both the present and future; his mind, admittedly, was not on the needs of disabled children, but few healthcare professionals would argue with the poet's fundamental hypothesis.

There is a growing literature on the history of services to disabled people in general (Davis 1997), and on the recent 'disability movement' (Barnes *et al.* 1999, Campbell and Oliver 1996) in particular, that may lead to a better understanding of both present services and their future development. The literature has included the emerging field of learning disability history, including the oral narratives of those who have lived through major upheavals in the 'care' meted out to them (Atkinson *et al.* 1997). The reader is presented here, however, with a broad overview of how Western societies from ancient times to the present have treated all those members they considered disabled, with the intention that this will provide the essential context to a study of existing provision, as well as a pointer to future developments.

It must be made clear at the outset that the study of disability history is complicated by the fact that records do not always distinguish one type of disability from another, and further, that the societies in question did not often see the need to discriminate between insanity, learning disability, sensory impairments or even dissidents in order to make provision for them (Winzer 1997).

Prehistoric societies

By definition, no records exist of how prehistoric societies treated their disabled members; but it is possible to surmise that in hunter-gatherer societies at least, it would be extraordinarily difficult for anyone with any sort of disability to survive such a nomadic and self-sufficient existence. We can only speculate as to the fate of less able members of such societies.

Ancient civilisations

Amongst the earliest literature referring to society's attitude towards disabled members are Hebrew writings, which suggest that those exhibiting bizarre behaviour were thought to be in the possession of evil spirits (Apter and Conoley 1984). The efforts of priests to exorcise these evil spirits frequently ended in the untimely demise of the patient.

The Ancient Egyptians were a little more enterprising, as well as generous. There is considerable evidence of their interest in treating the causes of disability, as well as social and educational provision for those with visual and intellectual impairments (Winzer 1997).

However, life was not so good for disabled people in the classical world. No less an intellectual than Aristotle decreed that no deformed child should be allowed to live, and in Sparta any infant considered unfit for citizenship or warrior status was either drowned or abandoned in the wilderness of the Taygetus mountains. For a period in Athens, disabled children were either killed or placed in clay pots by the roadside to die (Winzer 1997).

Significant improvements to the lot of disabled people arrived with the collapse of the Roman Empire and the advent of Christianity. Hospices were founded for those suffering from sensory impairments, intellectual and physical disabilities; indeed, legend has it that St Nicholas (now better known as Santa Claus) in his home town of Myra, provided accommodation for the retarded and dowries for poor girls (Barr 1913). But the church did not, then as now, speak with one voice. St Augustine of Hippo denied that the deaf were capable of faith, since they could not hear the word of the Lord, and also thought that epilepsy and insanity could only be cured by divine miracle (Winzer 1997).

Medieval period

The early medieval period saw no great breakthrough in society's provision for its less able members, generally considered butts for amusement. In sixteenth-century Hamburg, for example, learning-disabled people were confined in a tower in the city wall – known as the 'Idiot's Cage' (Winzer 1997). In England, conditions must have been better for those whose disabilities did not prevent them from assuming a viable role in the rural economy; and for those incapable of this, the enactment of the Poor Law in 1601 constituted the first attempt by the state to make provision for those disabled by poverty, mental or physical impairment. By this point, however, disability was firmly equated in the popular view with witchcraft, and the birth of an abnormal child was seen as proof of the parents' involvement in sinister practices – with the child itself enjoying the status of a changeling, or product of the Devil (Barnes *et al.* 1999).

The Renaissance

Perhaps the first real reforms to provision for disabled people came with the Renaissance, when serious studies of anatomy, surgery and medicine began in earnest. In Italy advances in the understanding of the anatomy of the ear made by those such as Bartlommeo Eustachio, led to a more thoughtful appreciation of individuals with impaired hearing, and the invention of the printing press, unsurprisingly, led to the first fumbling attempts to correct defective vision. Despite this progression, however, it was still possible for the German physician Paullini in 1698 to advocate beatings of the head for a range of conditions including epilepsy, paralysis, deafness, toothache and melancholia (Winzer 1997).

The 'lunatic' asylums

The early hospices for lunatics had catered besides for a wide variety of conditions that were by their very nature excluded from society – beggars, heretics, prostitutes, the unemployed and social dissidents found themselves incarcerated alongside the genuinely insane and retarded. The Hospital of St Mary of Bethlehem, established in 1247 and infamous later as 'Bedlam', saw the implementation of treatments based on the principle that 'Furious Mad-men are sooner, and more certainly cured by punishments, and hard usage, in a straight room, than by Physick or Medicines' (Winzer 1997). Most foundations were forced to become leprosariums until the leprosy epidemic subsided in the seventeenth century, by which time institutionalisation for all those falling into the very loosely defined category of the 'insane' was rife. The Industrial Revolution further reduced the contribution such members of society may have been able to make to their communities and increased the impact of their disability. But whilst they were conveniently tidied away from society, the inmates of Bedlam and similar hospitals were still considered objects of considerable entertainment, and spine-tingling tours of such provision were popular until the close of the nineteenth century (Winzer 1997).

Twentieth-century Britain

The early twentieth century in Britain saw the eventual categorisation of disabled people according to need, although the large class of 'mental defect-ives' still included those who were merely epileptic, and those considered morally suspect (Shanley and Starrs 1993). A distinction was also made between the 'aged and infirm', the insane and the mentally defective (Barnes *et al.* 1999). Learning-disabled people were classed (according to ability) under the 1913 Mental Deficiency Act as idiots, imbeciles or merely feeble-minded.

However, the basis of care remained the institution whether the unfortunate individual was physically or mentally disabled, had impaired hearing and/or vision or was mentally ill. Perhaps, partly as a result of hospital-based care, the 'medical' model of disability gained ground. Reinforced by the WHO definition of disability (see p. 14), this led to what has been termed the 'infantilisation' of disability (Barnes *et al.* 1999) and the creation of 'victim' roles for those affected. Notions of 'personal tragedy' affecting the families of disabled children, which still abound today (Glidden 1993) clearly stem from this ethos, which assumes that the disability is the individual's defining characteristic. Oliver has commented on the ramifications of this assumption, that 'personal tragedy theory has served to individualize the problems of disability and hence leave social and economic structures untouched' (Oliver 1996). The emphases of care were, and to some extent still are, very much upon diagnosis and predominantly medical treatment of individual disabilities.

Amongst the growing numbers of disabled people confined to institutions were a large proportion of children, who remained in hospital care until long after Jack Tizard's famous 'Brooklands' experiment in the 1950s. This experiment had involved the transfer of a number of children with severe learning disabilities, from an institution to a community group home, which demonstrated the intellectual, emotional and social benefits accruing to these children following their move (Tizard 1964). Yet it was not until the 1970s that a consortium of voluntary organisations led by Mencap and the Spastics Society, named EXODUS, took concerted action to move huge numbers of children out of hospital into small, local authority run homes. The effort was largely successful, although Baroness Jay reported in 1995 that there were still some children spending their lives in hospital, and others who were still admitted on a regular basis for respite care (Jay 1996).

In the meantime, conditions for adults institutionalised on the basis of their mental illness, learning or physical disability were not improving. On both sides of the Atlantic social scientists such as Goffman (1961) began to criticise 'asylums', and there was a growing realisation that institutional care for people with mental illnesses or learning disabilities was of its very nature vastly inadequate. Inherent in the 'asylum' approach were depersonalised care regimes, unsanitary living conditions and custodial models of care.

The fundamental assumption that hospital provision was in the best interests of those incarcerated was also stringently attacked. During the 1960s and 1970s in Britain, there was a spate of enquiries into the quality of 'care' being offered in hospitals to such 'patients' (as the ethos of the time dictated they were termed). The controversies raised by these enquiries drew much attention from the media. 'Subnormality' hospitals such as Borocourt (Jay 1996), Ely and Normansfield (Korman and Glennerster 1990) were subject to 'exposés' of their dehumanising and even abusive treatments. As late as 1981, a 'fly-on-the-wall' television documentary made in a couple of these hospitals included scenes of mental and physical abuse, and footage of a distressed and disruptive child tied to a pillar for the convenience of those around him (ATV 1981).

The impetus for change

The impetus for change came largely from the work of the social scientists mentioned above. In Britain this helped to fuel a more committed attitude on the part of government to achieving the social and political changes needed to deliver care to disabled people, which better respected their personhood.

Normalisation

This change in attitude was further stimulated by the writings and teachings of Wolf Wolfensberger, a Canadian social scientist who advocated the adoption of 'the normalisation principle' in approaches to any class of individuals devalued by society. His standard definition of normalisation runs thus:

> Utilization of means which are as culturally normative as possible, in order to establish and/or maintain personal behaviours and character-istics which are as culturally normative as possible
>
> (Wolfensberger 1972)

Initially this definition was adopted widely and enthusiastically, by profes-sionals, throughout the 1970s, but although articulated with the best of intentions, there are problems with such a definition as it has the potential to open the door to dangerous misinterpretations. It raises questions concern-ing *whose* norms are being used as the standard, and whether anyone has the right to impose their norms on anyone else. Wolfensberger's initial formula-tion of his ideas was soon under attack from many quarters (Emerson 1992). This led him to restate the principle as the concept of 'social role valorisa-tion', defined as 'The most explicit and highest goal of normalisation . . . the creation, support and defence of valued social roles for people who are at risk of devaluation' (Wolfensberger 1983).

The 'Five Service Accomplishments'

Whilst more acceptable on many grounds, the concept of social role valor-isation may seem difficult to translate into practice. This was left to John O'Brien, who in Britain translated Wolfensberger's principle into what have become widely known (and adopted by learning disability services) as the 'Five Service Accomplishments'. These require their subscribers to ensure that their service users are accorded:

- **Respect**, by offering users the chance to develop and maintain a positive image within their communities;
- **Community presence**, by providing living accommodation that is not only sited within a living community, but also which encourages partici-pation in that life;
- **Relationships** that are chosen by the individual, and that are lasting and meaningful to them;
- **Choice** in matters small (e.g. clothing) and large (e.g with whom or where to live)
- **Competence**, or at least the opportunity to learn and acquire skills and characteristics that have a positive effect on the individual's quality of life.

(O'Brien 1987)

Such has been the influence of O'Brien's service accomplishments that today it is rare to find a service for children with complex needs that does not include them in its underlying philosophy of care.

The right of choice

A crucial component of the Five Service Accomplishments is that of *choice* which was absent in Wolfensberger's original formulation of normalisation. It is only by exercising the right of choice that an individual can take control over his or her own life. Largely through strident campaigning over the past twenty years, the 'disability movement' has helped to contribute to society's grudging acknowledgement that its disabled members should be empowered to help themselves rather than accept a role of passive gratitude for any small concession meted out to them (Campbell and Oliver 1996). This, of course, applies as much to children with additional needs and their families as it does to disabled adults, and is reflected in recent guidelines on assessment (DoH 2000), as well as the recognition that families have a voice as authoritative as the professionals who attempt to meet their needs (Mencap1997; Russell 1997).

Children and choice

It is true, of course, that children have no legal right of consent, yet a growing amount of attention is being paid to the needs of children with complex needs to exert control and choice within their lives. Middleton (1999) has impressively articulated the rights of a disabled child *qua* child, rather than as 'proto-adult', and argued for the role of such children as agents of change both within their own lives, and in the broader political arena.

Whilst it cannot be denied that more conservative attitudes to the roles of disabled children exist, it must also be recognised that society has stumbled a long way from the belief that its infants with additional needs were the product of the Devil, or changelings. They may be tentative and timorous, but identifiable steps are now being taken towards such children enjoying the status of *agents* of change. It can only be hoped that this process continues, and that an awareness of the oppressive values and practices of the past informs a future for disabled children that allows them full citizenship and due control over their own lives.

References

Apter, S. J. and Conoley, J. C. (1984) *Childhood Behaviour Disorders and Emotional Disturbance*, Englewood Cliffs, N.J.: Prentice Hall.
Atkinson, D., Jackson, M. and Walmsley, J. (1997) *Forgotten Lives: Exploring the History of Learning Disability*, Kidderminster: British Institute of Learning Disabilities.
ATV (1981) *Silent Minority*, Television Documentary.

Barnes, C., Mercer, G. and Shakespeare, T. (1999) *Exploring Disability: A Sociological Introduction*, Cambridge: Polity Press.

Barr, M. (1913) *Mental defectives: Their history, treatment, and training*, Philadelphia: Blakiston.

Campbell, J. and Oliver, M. (1996) *Disability Politics: understanding our past, changing our future*, London, Routledge.

Davis, L. J. (1997) *The Disability Studies Reader*, London: Routledge.

Department of Health (1989) *The Children Act 1989: An Introductory Guide for the NHS*, London: Department of Health.

Department of Health (1995) *Disability Discrimination Act*, London: HMSO.

Department of Health (2000) *Framework for the Assessment of Children in Need*, London: DoH. (Also at www.doh.gov.uk/scg/cin.htm).

Emerson, E. (1992) 'What is normalisation?' in H. Brown and H. Smith (eds) *Normalisation: A Reader for the Nineties*, London: Routledge.

Glidden, L. M. (1993) 'What we do not know about families with children who have developmental disabilities: Questionnaire on Resources and Stress as a case study', *American Journal of Mental Retardation* 97, 481–495.

Goffman, E. (1961) *Asylum: Essays on the Social Situation of Mental Patients and Other Inmates*, New York: Doubleday.

Jay, P. (1996) 'EXODUS: Bringing Children Out of Hospital', in P. Mittler and V. Sinason (eds), *Changing Policy and Practice for People with Learning Disabilities*, London: Cassell.

Korman, N. and Glennerster, H. (1990) *Hospital Closure*, Milton Keynes: Open University Press.

Mencap (1997) *Left in the Dark: A Mencap report on the challenges facing the UK's 400,000 families of children with learning disability*, London: Mencap.

Middleton, L. (1999) *Disabled Children: Challenging Social Exclusion*, Oxford: Blackwell Science.

O'Brien, J. (1987) 'A guide to life planning: using the activities catalogue to integrate services and natural support systems', in B. W. Wilcox and G. T. Bellamy (eds) *The Activities Catalogue: an alternative curriculum for youth and adults with severe disabilities*, Baltimore: Brookes.

Oliver, M. (1992) 'Changing the Social Relations of Research Production?' *Disability, Handicap and Society* 7(2) 101–114.

Oliver, M. (1996) 'A Sociology of Disability or a Disablist Sociology?' in L. Barton (ed.) *Disability and Society: Emerging Issues and Insights*, London: Longman.

Rioux, M. and Bach, M. (eds) (1994) *Disability is not Measles: New Research Paradigms in Disability*, Ontario: Roeher Institute.

Russell, P. (1997) *Don't Forget Us: Children with Learning Disabilities and Severe Challenging Behaviour*, London: The Mental Health Foundation.

Shanley, E. and Starrs, T. A. (1993) *Learning Disabilities: A Handbook of Care*, London: Churchill Livingstone.

Swain, J., Finkelstein, V., French, S. and Oliver, M. (eds) (1997) *Disabling Barriers – Enabling Environments*, London: Sage Publications.

Tizard, J. (1964) *Community Services for the Mentally Handicapped*, Oxford: Oxford University Press.

UPIAS (1976) *Fundamental Principles of Disability*, London: Union of the Physically Impaired Against Segregation.

WHO (1980) *International Classification of Impairments, Disabilities and Handicaps*, Geneva: World Health Organisation.

Winzer, M. (1997) 'Disability and Society Before the Eighteenth Century', in L. J. Davis *The Disability Studies Reader*, London: Routledge.

Wolfensberger, W. (1972) *The Principle of Normalisation in Human Services*, Toronto: National Institute on Mental Retardation.

Wolfensberger, W. (1983) 'Social role valorization: A proposed new term for the principle of normalization', *Mental Retardation 21*, 234–239.

3   Challenging the 'tragedy'

Catherine Bernal

'I was told . . . that she'd be virtually a vegetable. The consultant virtually said you can lay her on the floor like a dog by the fire and she will not know anything or anybody, she'll be perfectly happy . . . it was all just such a shock because of what he said. Now it is totally different, she's got all emotions, and she is starting to do stepping and walking and things.'

(Mencap 1997: 8)

Assumptions of personal tragedy

This book is about the challenges involved in caring for children with complex disabilities, but evidence has shown consistently that one of the biggest stressors faced by these children's families is the assumption that the experience of having a child with severe disability is always a negative experience or unrelieved personal tragedy (Leonard 1999; Mencap 1997). This assumption, made both by society at large and by some professionals in particular, may be detected in many forms. Sometimes even well-intentioned support groups have perpetuated this assumption, for example, the logo of the sad little child (nicknamed 'Little Joey') that was adopted by Mencap until recently.

Researchers have been accused of 'pathologising' families by their assumptions of trauma (Glidden 1993) whilst neglecting the more rewarding aspects of parenting a child with a disability. Professionals giving the news of a child's newly diagnosed disability to the parents may unwittingly reinforce this view. 'I'm sorry to say your child has Down's syndrome' (Leonard 1999: 15) is typical of many communications received by new parents. This process has been termed by one prominent author on the subject 'abnormalisation', or 'the creation of special need' (Middleton 1999).

It could be suggested that whilst such a widespread attitude may inspire the public to give generously to those they perceive to be in need, it is perhaps not so helpful to the individual child and his or her family. This 'tragedy' model is supported by what has already been described as the 'medical' model of disability (Chapter 2), which imposes a limit on individual potential and gives professionals the right to exercise their expertise, often at the cost to the family's self-determination (Case 2000). Perhaps the most serious consequence, however, of this perception of the family's being stricken by tragedy is that it does not help the parents to adjust to their child's disability, or develop the confidence to cope. Instead the parents are encouraged to feel isolated and disempowered by their status as victims of a catastrophe (Leonard 1999). A further danger of this attitude is that the professional's corresponding rush of sympathy – in place of empathy – will do little to build a productive relationship with the family they are intending to support (Stein-Parbury 1993).

Finally, the child is necessarily devalued alongside his or her potential (Middleton 1999) for development. Explicit within the United Nations Convention on the Rights of the Child (Morris 1998) is the individual's rights for inclusion, development and freedom of expression. It is only when a social model of disability has been adopted by all in contact with the child that these rights can be met. This cannot happen whilst the child is seen as the 'victim' of a tragedy.

Challenging

It must be emphasised, however, that this chapter is not an attempt to deny the grief (or 'chronic sorrow'), frustration and pain that almost invariably accompany the experience of giving birth to and bringing up a disabled child. Such emotions are not uncommon (Dale 1996), but their identification need not lead to assumptions of persistent grief for the parents and catastrophe for the child. Here, therefore, we present some of the evidence to the contrary, hoping to demonstrate that there can be positive aspects to parenting a disabled child, and it is important that every professional involved with such families should be as conscious of the possible positive aspects as they are of the possible costs to family life.

Sadly, there has been little research into the positive aspects of parenting a disabled child, and it is only comparatively recently in the study of disability that attention has shifted onto this arena of experience. Seligman and Darling (1989) reported that

> the tremendous adaptive capacity of families is evidenced by the fact that given all the obstacles to the parent–child attachment present in the case of childhood disability, the vast majority do form strong attachments to their disabled infants.

They also emphasise that different families will react differently on the basis of psychological, material and socio-economic factors (Seligman and Darling 1989). Research by Scope found that most of the parents of disabled children interviewed stated that love for and pride in their children far outweighed any distress related to them (Leonard 1999).

As a result of a longitudinal study of families with a disabled member, Beresford (1994) was able to report that parents did not see their child as a disabled person, but as an individual with particular challenges and restrictions stemming from their physical impairment. The words of the parents themselves will form a large part of the remainder of this chapter.

Although there is considerable literature on negative parental reactions following the diagnosis of disability in their child, some have been known to respond positively to the news. Dale (1996: 68) reports one mother's relief when she announced to her uncomprehending health visitor,

> 'Well, thank God, he's only got Down's syndrome. It could be worse.'

Another parent, whose baby had just survived the first few days of an uncertain life, reacted violently to her social worker's suggestion that she must be grieving for the perfect child she had wanted,

> 'Grieving? Bereaved? . . . I'm over the moon; we had thought we had lost her.'
>
> (Leonard 1999: 18)

Contrary to popular belief, dissatisfaction with the manner of professional communication of the news has been demonstrated to be unrelated to perceptions of tragedy; which suggests that even at this stage, parents can have a balanced view of their child's potential (Cunningham *et al*. 1984).

Childhood disability often manifests itself in ways that are, to society at large, unattractive and stigmatising. Case (2000), however, found that when descriptions of their children's appearance were solicited, the majority of parents gave images in which their offspring appeared attractive, contented, sociable and bright. Beresford (1994: 62), too, encountered many positive descriptions by parents of their child, including the following:

> 'A lot of people have said how appealing he is and what a nice child he is. It's like a lot of special children they've got their own sort of beauty.'

Case (2000) also reported that the affected children in his study both sought and returned affection readily, with few signs of anti-social behaviour. This apparently common characteristic perhaps makes it easier for parents to accept their child's disability and bond with the infant in a very normal way:

> '. . . perhaps some parents would give up the baby – but I wouldn't have . . . I wouldn't give her up for the world . . .'
>
> (Leonard 1999: 14)

The parents interviewed by Beresford's team often reported their child's sense of humour in appreciative terms. One mother said of her child with Down's syndrome:

'She's very, very comical. She loves to play and laugh and joke. She loves to sing and dance. She gives a great deal of pleasure to everybody around her in that way. She'll have the whole room laughing. Although she has got problems, she has still brought into our world the joy that any other child would bring and more.'

(Beresford 1994: 62)

A consequence of the children's readiness to give and receive affection, as well as their sense of humour, is often a highly positive relationship with their parents (Beresford 1994; Case 2000). One parent commented:

'We share a lot of giggles. She's got quite a sense of humour and it's very easy to say the right things to trigger that off, and that brings us closer.'

(Beresford 1994: 63)

It is this quality of relationship, of course, that allows parents to 'keep going' and to continue to see the positive side of their parenting experience; a circular and deeply satisfying effect for those who encounter it. Sometimes, however, when a child's needs can be sufficiently great to warrant either respite or permanent residential care, the distance from the parent can improve the relationship and help the latter to focus on the more positive aspects of the child:

'Having some distance from Chrissy has altered my perspectives; I now value her more. She has a great sense of humour and we often giggle together over silly-sounding words. She loves hugs and kisses and has a smile that lights up her face. I never appreciated her uniqueness as I do now.'

(Gregory 2000)

The positive aspects of parenting a child with a disability have been presented here not just as a point of interest, but also because parents' abilities to adjust to life with the child will only be aided by professional avoidance of preconceived notions of 'tragedy' and its replacement by true recognition of the complete range of experiences that follow a diagnosis of disability. As Case (2000) boldly states, 'parents with disabled children must be given equal rights in society, and have their positive experiences highlighted, elaborated and celebrated'. Whilst not wishing to devalue the negative aspects of the whole experience, we hope here to have gone some way towards redressing the balance – and that a more sensitive approach to parents of the disabled child in hospital will result.

References

Beresford, B. (1994) *Positively Parents: Caring for a Severely Disabled Child*, York: Social Policy Research Unit.

Case, S. (2000) 'Refocusing on the Parent: what are the social issues of concern for parents of disabled children?' *Disability and Society*, 15(2): 271–292.

Cunningham, C. C, Morgan, P. A. and McGucken, R. B. (1984) 'Down's Sydrome: is dissatisfaction with diagnosis inevitable?' *Developmental Medicine and Child Neurology*, 26(1) 33–39.

Dale, N. (1996) *Working with Families of Children with Special Needs: Partnership and Practice*, London: Routledge.

Glidden, L. M. (1993) 'What We Do *Not* Know About Families With Children Who Have Developmental Disabilities: Questionnaire on Resources and Stress as a Case Study', *American Journal on Mental Retardation*, 97(5) 481–495.

Gregory, J. (2000) *Bringing up a challenging child: When love is not enough*, London: Jessica Kingsley.

Leonard, A. (1999) *Right from the Start: Looking at diagnosis and disclosure – parents describe how they found out about their child's disability*, London: Scope.

Mencap (1997) *Left in the Dark: a Mencap report on the challenges facing the UK's 400,000 families of children with learning disabilities*, London: Mencap.

Middleton, L. (1999) *Disabled Children: Challenging Social Exclusion*, Oxford: Blackwell.

Morris, J. (1998) *Accessing Human Rights: Disabled children and the Children Act*, Ilford: Barnado's.

Seligman, M. and Darling, R. B. (1989) *Ordinary Families, Special Children: A System Approach to Childhood Disability*, New York: Guilford Press.

Stein-Parbury, J. (1993) *Patient and Person: Developing interpersonal skills in nursing*, London: Churchill Livingstone.

4 Ethics: rationing healthcare and resources

Kim Broster

Introduction

In a time of prioritising services and targeting client populations, this chapter explores the sometimes conflicting ethics that underpin the decision-making process in relation to the allocation of services for children with disabilities. It concludes that the two major perspectives, utilitarianism and deontology, whilst having different underlying principles, both reach an ethical conclusion that the child with special needs is equally deserving of services as the child without a disability.

Some of the issues for discussion are encapsulated in the following quotation from a telephone call received at the local Children's Centre, where services for children with disabilities are delivered and coordinated. The Health Visitor sounding exasperated asked the following question: 'I've got a number of children on my case load who I have referred for Speech and Language Therapy, they have been placed on a waiting list for the next year. Why is it that the children with the most complex needs and poorer prognosis are seen immediately and the Early Intervention Therapy Team has dedicated speech therapist time, while the children I have referred who I believe have a much better chance of benefiting from this input have to wait?'

What is interesting about this statement is that the Health Visitor appeared to be making a value judgement on which children should or could most benefit from the allocation of services in her view. What was not implied was that all children should have equal access. This raises the question of whether the allocation of services is about duty of care or prioritising finite resources.

There is an assumption that the predominant underlying philosophy, which runs throughout the health service, is that of utilitarianism i.e. endeavouring to achieve the greatest all round good for all concerned within the care of any individual patient. One of the original utilitarians, Jeremy Bentham (1748–1832) defined it in these terms:

> Utilitarianism is what tends to produce, benefit, or advance pleasure, good or happiness, either for the individual or for the community. The good of the greatest number is the criterion of right or wrong.

However, it is possible to distinguish other different purposes or aims for services, for example human rights, utilitarian and clinical. The future development of services continues to depend upon which of these aims the NHS decides to sign up to.

With the human rights issue it is often claimed that the aim of services is to enable individuals to make better informed decisions about their own health, for example, to change their lifestyle or to accept or refuse treatment. In the case of the child with disability, however, treatment is often not concerned with cure but with preventing further complications or ensuring that the child can achieve their full potential. This approach is viewed as problematic as the choices of individuals' impact upon others. This has always been true of the health service, where finite resources have meant that for every decision to treat there is an opportunity cost. An example of this is where some more recent innovations in clinical treatment may be denied the child with disability.

Within the utilitarian approach to the delivery of healthcare the aim of many health programmes is to reduce the prevalence of the disease in the community or population as a whole. For example the recent research into genetics has meant that while it may provide an important major step towards enabling people to make genuinely free decisions about their future reproduction, or to improve the support and services for people with disabilities, the screening out of any disabling conditions could have consequences for the value which society places on the life of the individual with a disability, such as the debate that surrounds the parent who decides to go ahead with a pregnancy where the baby is known to have a disabling condition.

Clinical issues surrounding best treatment for the individual patient may not take into account the needs of society as a whole or in some circumstances a clinician may only carry out a test or screening programme if there is something 'clinically valid' which can be done with the information. This can impede research or, as stated before, exempt some individuals from being considered for a new treatment.

One of the most fundamental questions is, what do patients, health professionals, and government understand by the concept of valid? Some purchasers and clinicians may be unwilling to spend money on a service that only provides an individual with more information about their future health status in the absence of any clinical intervention, and may prefer to invest in services, which are known to improve the health status of the population. Therefore, conflicts arise when questioning whose interests are paramount, those of the child, the parents, health professionals or society.

Followers of Kant (the 17th-century philosopher cited in Rumbould 1993), known as deontologists, would claim that the decision should be made in terms of 'duty' and that intrinsically the right or wrong of a decision would be clear if the consequences of such a decision were to imply harm. 'Good behaviour is self-justifying, bad behaviour is self-condemning: no other supporting evidence is required'. Denying treatment to the child with disability could therefore be construed as self-condemning. According to Rumbould (1993) the Kantian viewpoint is less clear, often requiring individuals to 'exercise' their reason to arrive at a 'logically sound maxim'. Thus individuals are to some extent left to decide for themselves what their duty is, which could cause conflict. However, the issue here has been clouded by the prioritisation of finite resources, so that the utilitarianism of 'greatest happiness principle' comes into play. If the ends justify the means and denying treatment to one group of children means that another larger group benefit, this for some may be justification. However the basic problem with this argument is deciding who are the judge and jury on who should receive the services.

In the question from the Health Visitor that opened this chapter, there was an assumption that one group was suffering at the expense of another: underlying this was an assumption that one group, the child without major special needs/disability was somehow more deserving. In an essay regarding ethical issues in the care of a profoundly multi-handicapped child, Philip Darbyshire (1986) raises the important ethical issue of the humanity or personhood of the profoundly disabled child, and asks the controversial question, is such a child really a human or person in any sense of the word? If a society considers that the basis of personhood is characterised by the level of a person's IQ or what they can give back to the society in which they live, how is the child with disability judged?

It is difficult to imagine a situation in which nurses could comfortably work within an ethical framework, which viewed a profoundly disabled child as a non-person. We have only to look to history and Nazi Germany to see what can happen when disabled people are viewed as less than human. Today it is generally accepted that a social role is taken and the child with profound disabilities is viewed as a child first and foremost. However, it is important to remember that in childhood, functional disability very much relates to age and that the disability may become more pronounced with age.

Every parent has expectations of their children. Initially the extent of the impairment is often unclear. No one can predict a child's future ability and indeed the provision of services and equipment depend on optimism rather than complacency.

Relating severity of disability to needs can be difficult. Within a medical model this might seem possible if we knew enough about impairments, their origin, classification and severity. In practice this is not the case and the child's needs are therefore something which is discerned in relationship to the abilities of the developing child and not, as when it is used in adult life, to the static model of an 'able' adult.

Inasmuch as we can be objective about disability there is still a problem because of its poor correlation with role disadvantage (handicap in the medical model). This is because a major component of role disadvantage is environmental and best described in a social model. The most common practical approach is to define disadvantage by the level of need. This is thought to be useful because as service providers it is the level of need that causes most concern. The pitfall is that provision is not a reliable measure of need and unmet needs are rarely recorded.

There is a 'duty' of care that is clear in both professional codes of conduct and in law. Beneficence and non-maleficence are cited within the code of professional conduct produced by NMC (2002), 'the nurse shall act always in such a way as to promote and safeguard the well-being and interests of patients/clients and . . . they shall ensure that no action or omission on his her part or within his/her sphere of influence is detrimental to the condition or safety of patients/carers'.

The Children Act (1989) lays a duty upon local authorities to provide services designed to minimise the effects of impairments upon children and to help them lead as full lives as possible. There has been a move away from institutional care towards community care with regard to children with disability; children used to be cared for in long-term children's hospitals without education or any real treatment apart from care.

The UN Convention on the Rights of the Child, which was ratified by the Government in December 1991, recognises that children are a vulnerable group entitled to special care and assistance. It sets out the principles to be taken into account in any legislation, policy and practice, which impacts on children.

Kopelman (1984) describes three main reasons why children with profound disabilities are owed our respect:

> Firstly they have the ability to feel. Secondly, how they are treated affects our institutions; thus it is in our own self-interests to see that they are treated respectfully. Third, we share our communities and homes with them; we respect the commitment, benevolent concern or affection that holds families and communities together.

Beardshaw (1981) described the poor quality of care that can result when care staff come to accept that the individuals in their care are somehow less than persons or less than human. There is a need to see these children not as permanently lacking in essential attributes but as being primarily children with a capacity for development however limited that may be.

There are other important ethical principles, such as respect for persons and their autonomy. If autonomy is accepted as a valuable ethical principle then nurses will want to consider ways in which they might increase the autonomy for the child with profoundly disabling conditions. There are issues related to privacy, respect for human dignity and integrity and the commitment of nursing to treat children as individuals. This could be applied to trying not to place limits on a child's autonomy and their right to the level of independence they may be capable of achieving however minimal this might be. There is the principle of justice, which incorporates the ideals

of fairness, equality and non-discrimination. This often tends to be discussed in relation to larger issues, such as the allocation of resources but, it
should be remembered that the health professional's time and care is one of
the most valuable of resources.

Therefore, the ethical self-awareness of the health professional is most
pivotal in the delivery of appropriate care. Further, when the care of children
with disabilities is evaluated, it should be in terms of how their development
has been encouraged, how individualised their care has been and how they
have been helped to integrate with the community at large.

Positive outcomes can also be measured in how they have been involved in
pleasurable experiences and how they have been helped to stay in the best
possible physical and nutritional condition. Also important is how they have
been communicated with and had their attempts at communication attended
to. Also how they have been generally loved and cared for. This in essence is
the 'moral sense of nursing' described by Bishop and Scudder (1987) who
suggest that 'children at their most vulnerable and dependent have every
right to expect this of us'. This can also be related to the 'greatest happiness'
principal.

One of the problems that face managers in the NHS is that there are no
clear guidelines as to what is an acceptable level of provision; this is as true
of the level of services dedicated to children with disabilities as it is of the
provision of surgical beds. Attempts to set standards are debated both
locally and nationally and there is what has been termed a 'postcode lottery'
when it comes to the level of services received. Areas vary tremendously in
the services they provide and by whom, with some areas having a higher
percentage of educational-funded services, or voluntary-funded places e.g.
by SCOPE or MENCAP. Jo Lenaghan in *Rationing and Rights in Health Care*,
(1996) suggests that responsibilities may be distributed as follows:

- The government should decide what services the NHS should provide.
- Health authorities should decide on the level of services to be provided.
- Clinicians should decide which individuals to give priority to, according
  to the framework set by government.
- The public should be involved in debates about what services should
  be provided and should have the opportunity to challenge unfair
  decisions.

However, if this is to happen the debate has to be open, honest and ethical.
This includes honest discussion about the value base of decisions taken by
government regarding the allocation of resources and how 'needs' are
assessed. There also needs to be honest discussion about whether the rationing of resources is to reduce expenditure or due to a lack of qualified staff
and training places.

In conclusion, both the following major ethical principles can be applied
to the child with disability and arguments taken from both that endorse the

ethical imperative that treatment to the child with disability is never denied. First, from the Kantian philosophy: that it is intrinsically wrong to do harm and to make judgement on the value of an individuals quality of life based on what they can do for society. Second, a utilitarian approach that society as a whole, if it is agreed that society can be judged by the actions it takes, loses out if care of a vulnerable group is deemed unnecessary.

Children with disability deserve our care, this can be based on the moral principles of beneficence, justice and respect for persons, but also as children who have an extraordinary need to be valued for what they are and for what they may yet become.

References

Beardshaw, V. (1981) 'Conscientious Objectors at Work: Mental hospital nurses – a case study' in G. Brykczynska (ed.) *Ethics in Paediatric Nursing*; London: Chapman and Hall.

Bentham, J. (1748–1832) cited in *Ends and means II: Mill and Utilitarianism*.

Bishop, A. H. and Scudder, J. R. Jnr. (1987) 'Nursing ethics in an age of controversy', *Journal of Advanced Nursing Science* 9 (3): 34–43.

Children Act (1989) London: HMSO.

Darbyshire, P. (1986) *Ethical issues in the care of the profoundly multiply-handicapped child*, Chapter 6 in G. Brykczynska (ed.) *Ethics in Paediatric Nursing*, London: Chapman and Hall.

Lenaghan, J. (1996) *Rationing and Rights in Healthcare*, London: IPPR.

Kopelman, L. (1984) 'Respect and the retarded: issues of valuing and labelling', in L. Kopelman and J. C. Moskop (eds) *Ethics and Mental Retardation*, Dordrecht: D. Reidel/Kluwer.

Nursing and Midwifery Council (2002) *Code of Professional Conduct* London: NMC.

Rumbould, G. (1993) *Ethics in Nursing Practice*, London: Balliere Tindall.

UN *Convention on the Rights Of the Child* (1991) London: HMSO.

Further reading

Brykczynska, G. (1992) *Ethics in Paediatric Nursing*, London: Chapman and Hall.

Dale, N. (1996) *Working with Families of Children with Special Needs*, London: Routledge.

Dracopoulou, S. (1998) *Ethics and Values in Healthcare Management*, London: Routledge.

Hunter, D. J. (1997) *Desperately Seeking Solutions Rationing Healthcare*, New York: Longman.

Lenaghan, J. (1996) *Rationing and Rights in Healthcare*, London: IPPR.

Lenaghan, J. (1998) *Brave New NHS? The impact of the new genetics on the health service*, London: IPPR.

5   Getting it right – the initial diagnosis

Kim Broster and Helen K. Warner

One of the most momentous events for a family is learning about their child's disability. This may occur prior to the birth, at birth, or even several years later. Parents tend to express greater dissatisfaction regarding how they were informed of the disability than with almost any other interactions regarding their children (Russell 1991). This chapter reviews current research that shows that the way in which the diagnosis is given can have a beneficial effect on subsequent parent-child relationships and the relationship between parents and professionals. It concludes with guidelines for implementing a policy for best practice regarding the giving of a diagnosis to the parents of children with long-term special needs.

Significant issues regarding the initial diagnosis of disability, have been defined by Cunningham and Davis (1985), who describe how the criticisms voiced by parents fall into three categories as follows:

> *The manner of the person giving the diagnosis*: This may be unsympathetic, cold, insensitive, and expressed in language too difficult or vague to understand.
> *Problems with information*: There may be a lack of information and guidance about the diagnosis and what can be done. The information may be highly negative, often misleading, contradictory and inaccurate. Information may be denied altogether. Conversely too much information can be overwhelming.
> *Organisational aspects*: There may be a delay and difficulty in getting access to help; there may also be a lack of privacy and a lack of co-ordination between services.

Whilst there are many examples of models of good practice in relation to the giving of a diagnosis, it would appear that the lack of implementation of these is mainly due to the belief that there is little one can do to improve the situation, 'there is no good way to tell bad news' and people will always react angrily to 'the bearer of such news'. In 1977 doctors were reportedly unwilling to admit they had told patients badly; such criticisms are inevitable and stem from resentment at the diagnosis. In more recent literature, there remain too many examples of insensitive professionals with negative attitudes towards the disabled, and shocking stories of poor treatment (St John 2004).

It is often suggested that parents' recollections are inaccurate as they are confused at the moment of emotional upset. It is also well documented that many parents find it difficult to assimilate the information given to them at the time of diagnosis but this should only offer further justification for following aspects of good practice concerned with giving time and further opportunities to discuss the diagnosis. Most parents do remember aspects of the disclosure in vivid detail, e.g. 'flashbulb' memories. McConachie (1990) discusses the feelings of isolation as parents have to deal with other people's reactions to the news and are pressured to 'cope'.

There is growing evidence that the way in which parents are told the news affects how they adjust to the situation and their subsequent treatment of the child. Therefore, it is extremely important that this is recognised. In a land-mark study, Cunningham *et al.* (1984) interviewed 62 sets of parents who had babies with Down's syndrome, identified at birth. Of these sets 58 per cent expressed some form of dissatisfaction with the timing or manner of telling. A 'model procedure' was then instituted in one health authority based on current best practice. In contrast to previous practice, all the parents who were informed using the new procedure registered satisfaction. Moreover, they showed positive attitudes towards their child, themselves and their ongoing professional services and help six months later.

In a further study, Quinne and Rutter (1994) interviewed 166 mothers of children with severe learning disabilities around the time of their initial diagnosis. They were asked to rate the doctor's affective behaviour and their understanding and memory of the information they received. Measures were also included to take account of the child's age when the diagnosis was made and how satisfied they were with the way in which they were told the diagnosis. Similarly to other studies, 58 per cent of parents reported dissatis-faction with the communication. Satisfaction was found to be much higher if the person communicating the diagnostic information was perceived as having a sympathetic manner, being direct and approachable, showing understanding of the mother's concern, and being a good communicator.

A main communication task during the diagnostic period is to communi-cate information about the child's condition and special needs to the parents in terms that can be understood and remembered. This will enable the parent to start adjusting to the reality of the child's condition and some of its potential consequences and future prognosis. In the words of the President of the Royal College of Paediatrics and Child Health 2000–2003, Professor Sir David Hall, ' . . . conveying difficult news to parents is just as much of an art form as doing an operation and it's just as important to be self-critical' (*Right From the Start Template* 2003). Sharing the news with at least one other professional enables Professor Sir David Hall and colleagues to debrief, learning and reflecting together after the event.

The above evidence shows that good disclosure practice prevents much distress for parents, fosters good parent-professional relationships, facilitates the attachment process and early care for the child and, when incorporated with family support services over the first years, reduces levels of anxiety and stress.

The requirements for any policy must take into account the need for privacy, giving a balanced view with timely information, while ensuring that the parent is supported. Questions need to be answered honestly and with written information to follow. Having a policy in place is not enough, however, and there is a requirement for all staff to assist with its implementation. In the research, great emphasis is placed on the importance the parent attributes to the manner of the 'teller' and this aspect of any policy will need to be supported by training for staff as it is perhaps the most difficult to implement.

It is essential that there is a named professional who takes the responsibility for ensuring that good practice is carried out. This professional should have access to audit from several sources, including parent support groups and 'befriending schemes' in addition to the more formal audit of individual interviews or questionnaires.

Although relevant for professionals, the policy initiative *Together From The Start* (2003), has been criticised for not addressing the emotional wellbeing of families where there is a child with a learning disability (St John 2004). Counselling may be spoken of in passing by doctors or other professionals but few parents may initiate looking for counselling when their time is already taken up with many other appointments. However, if counselling is available and accessible and there is some understanding of the particular stresses faced by parents of children with special needs, there is considerable demand and many parents have found this to be beneficial (Shampan 2002). Although this will initially be about the diagnosis and expectations, it is likely that further work will be necessary throughout the child's life at times of transition, as new hurdles arise for the family (Bicknell 1983). As the child grows into a young person they may be particularly vulnerable to adjustment difficulties as they come to realise their limitations in contrast to their siblings and peers (Royal College of Psychiatrists 2004). Families often require help to understand their child's behaviour; facilitation of their developing parenting skills; enhancement of their coping mechanisms; and help to promote appropriate play, occupation and communication (Royal College of Psychiatrists 2004).

It would appear, however, that rather than seeking professional counselling, parents are more likely to bring their concerns to professionals who are already directly working with their children and with whom they have established a relationship. In such instances when parents react to events with anger, denial and sadness, the professional is required to be non-defensive, and help the parent to progress to a mature emotional acceptance of the child and his/her disability. In order for a productive partnership with parents to develop, genuineness, respect and empathy are required, as suggested by

Rogers (1980). Parents need professionals to be optimistic but objective about their child's development and to facilitate a problem-solving approach.

Basic counselling and listening skills are therefore vital. The term 'counselling' refers to any situation between two people in which one construes the other as having the relevant competence and willingness to assist, and the other has the intention to do so. Therefore counselling occurs when the speech and language therapist communicates the results of a language assessment, or the occupational therapist advises on a mobility aid. It might be potentially more dramatic when the paediatrician is communicating a severe diagnosis, but the skills required remain the same. Many of these skills, it can be argued, are basic to social interaction. However professionals may lack confidence in using them, or may be unaware of the counselling process. They may also construe that they should act differently in a professional capacity as compared to a personal situation. It would therefore seem essential that all healthcare professionals undertake compulsory basic counselling skills training and that it is included in their job description.

McGonigal *et al.* (1991) asserted that an enabling approach to family work requires professionals to re-examine traditional roles and practices, and develop new ones which promote mutual respect and partnership. The focus of change should be on parent-professional partnership. However, Cunningham and Davis (1985) suggest that partnership working is also extended to professionals, each member bringing his/her own expertise and complementary skills and having equal status in the team.

The early years of learning are critically important and when targeted they can maximise the learning potential of children. Early intervention following the diagnosis is therefore vital. The transdisciplinary model was specifically developed to address the principles of family-centred, early intervention, in the belief that the child's development in the physical, cognitive, and social domains is interdependent and complex. Doyle (1997) summarised this approach as follows:

- Different disciplinary perspectives are embedded in an ecological perspective on the child within his/her family to produce a complex but relevant development picture.
- Such an integrated approach should be free of professional contradictions and therefore of confusion.
- The emphasis on the child within the family context is more meaningful to parents and potentially more empowering.
- The process allows for significant professional development (explaining your own perspective deepens knowledge and understanding and so does understanding another perspective. The potential for effectiveness is also increased).

Each discipline has a piece of the puzzle and it is only when they all come together that the full picture can be seen. Warner (2001) describes her endeavours to implement this way of working within a child development centre, and some of the difficulties encountered.

It could be argued that the transdisciplinary model of working is a precursor of the person-centred planning approach that is advocated as the child becomes a young person, and begins to think of his/her future needs together with their friends, family and professionals involved. Sanderson (2004) takes this a step further and describes essential family lifestyle plans to ensure the whole family's needs can be met, and not just those of the disabled person to the detriment of other family members. The transdisciplinary model is a way of creating a 'team around the child' to include parents, as experts in their own right, and professionals. Regular meetings allow for information sharing, goal reviewing and the setting of new goals. It is mutually supportive, enabling parents to see the whole team united in wanting the best for their child, as well as being accessible to answer questions and respond to any concerns.

Limbrick's (2001) 'Team around the Child' Model has evolved in recent years due to the widely perceived need for an integrated approach within existing resources. In this model the keyworker co-ordinates the services, acting as the 'interface' between the individual family and all local services. The benefits include the family having a supportive team with whom they can discuss their child's and family's needs and the professionals being able to mutually support each other instead of feeling isolated and unsupported in their work. This way of working, in the same way as the transdisciplinary model, allows the child and parents to prioritise goals and not feel overloaded or confused by conflicting advice from practitioners working alone. Such integrated or holistic goals recognise that children do not function in a discipline-specific way and so will appear more relevant to parents, and will also be motivating to the child (Limbrick 2003).

An integrated pathway, based on the 'team around the child' model, and described by Limbrick (2003), reflects the collaboration between agencies, services and practitioners and a seamless and responsive service for children and their families. The ideal is described as a 'single all-embracing multi-agency pathway' although it is acknowledged that it may take many years to achieve this.

Professional support from the beginning provides a safety net at a time of uncertainty, but the reality is that many parents end up feeling angry towards professionals due to difficulties in accessing help (St John 2004). Relationships between partners can also become strained following a diagnosis, and there is still too little provision for supporting fathers. Many assessments may be made and needs identified, but relevant interventions for the child and family do not always happen as a result.

Conclusion

Parents' reactions to the news that their child has a disability will vary according to their previous experiences, and their interactions with other people before, during and after the time the news is received. The meanings they attach to their child's disability will continue to change as the child grows and they encounter new situations.

There should be compulsory basic listening or counselling skills training programmes for all professionals included in their job descriptions, so that conflict of interest may be avoided. Emotional support should be identified for the family at an early stage to promote adaptation to their new situation, attachment to the child, and to foster a good relationship with professionals. Considering the needs of the family in the context of the individual experi-ence of family members will enhance their ability to deal with the impact of this potentially life changing event. Professionals who are already directly involved with the child and family will be best placed to offer this kind of support. If they also have the opportunity to debrief and reflect on their practice, they will continue to learn from it. Clinical supervision provides a forum for this reflection, for both self-criticism and acknowledgement of good practice to take place, and this will enhance both personal and profes-sional development.

In practice, however, although research has consistently demonstrated the importance of these wider-ranging factors and their importance to long-term outcomes for children with disabilities and their families, assessment often continues to focus on child developmental levels only.

Recommendations

- Review local policies regarding training of medical and nursing staff.
- Revisit with staff the importance of sensitive and timely disclosure.
- Update local policy.
- Allocate the implementation and audit of the policy to a named professional.

A policy on guidelines for giving a diagnosis of disability should include the following considerations:

1   The diagnosis should be given by a consultant paediatrician and where ever possible with a specialist Health Visitor or suitably qualified mem-ber of nursing staff.
2   The diagnosis should be given as soon as possible, except in cases of maternal ill health. If the exact diagnosis is not known this should not deter staff from giving honest answers when they suspect that something is wrong.
3   The diagnosis should be given to both parents together whenever pos-sible. In the case of a single parent a family member or friend should also be present. Other relatives should be allowed to be present where this is requested. An interpreter should be present where the parent is not fluent in English.

4   A diagnosis should be given in privacy and be undisturbed.
5   Wherever possible the diagnosis should be given with the baby or young child present. Exceptions would be for the critically ill child or an older child who may need to be informed with parents on a separate occasion.
6   Diagnosis should be given directly, with time for the parents to ask questions. A balanced viewpoint should be transmitted.
7   Diagnosis should be given with a sympathetic, caring and humane attitude, taking account of the parent's emotional state and ability to take in verbal information.
8   An arrangement should be made for the Specialist Health Visitor or another key person to see the parents as soon as they are ready, and a contact telephone number given.
9   Parents should have the opportunity to remain alone in a private place for as long as they need.
10 Diagnosis needs to be followed up with a written summary of what has been discussed along with a follow-up appointment.
11 Information should be given where possible of how the parent may arrange to speak to another parent of a child with a similar disability or a parent support scheme

Most of these guidelines are to be found in the RCN Guidelines (1999) and the document *Together from the start – practical guidance for professionals working with disabled children and their families* (2003), which was produced by a multi-agency working party for the Department of Education and Skills and the Department of Health, www.rightfromthestart.org.uk
   Follow-up for each family should include:

*   An offer to talk to other family members or advice given on how to cope with other people's reactions.
*   Further opportunities to go over the initial information.
*   Supportive counselling offered in the parent's own home.
*   Information on benefits and services.
*   Introduction of other services as appropriate.
*   Appointing of a key worker.

There is also a training handbook and video entitled *Giving, Hearing and Living with the News of a Child's Disability*, ISBN 1 898244 391.
   Contact: www.learningdisabilities.org.uk to obtain a copy of *First Impressions: Emotional and Practical Support for Families* by Alison Cowan, from the Foundation for People with Learning Disabilities.

Further reading

Bicknell, J. (1983) 'The psychopathology of handicap', *British Journal of Medical Psychology* 56,167–178.

Cunningham, C. C. and Davis, H. (1985) *Working with Parents: Frameworks for Collaboration*, Milton Keynes: Open University Press.

Cunningham C. C., Morgan P. A. and McGucken R. B. (1984) 'Down's Syndrome: is dissatisfaction with disclosure of diagnosis inevitable?' *Developmental Medicine and Child Neurology*; 26, 33–39.

Dale, N. (1997) *Working with Families of Children with Special Needs*, London: Routledge.

Davis, H. (1993) *Counselling Parents of Children with Chronic Illness or Disability*: Leicester: BPS Books.

Department of Education and Skills (2003) *Together from the Start – Practical guidance for professionals working with Disabled Children and their Families*, London: HMSO.

Department of Health, Scope (2003) *Right From The Start Template: Good practice in sharing the news*, DoH: Scope in partnership with the Right From The Start Working Group.

Doyle, B. (1997) 'Transdisciplinary approaches to working with families', in B. Carpenter (ed.) *Families in Context: Emerging Trends in Family Support and Early Intervention*, London: Fulton.

Freeman, M. (1999) 'Can different healthcare professionals really work as a team?', *Nursing Management* 6(7) 10–13.

Harris, S. (1987) *Early Intervention for children with motor handicaps: The effectiveness of Early Intervention for at-risk and handicapped children*, Orlando, Fla: Academic Press.

Hornby, G. (1994) *Counselling in Child Disability*, London: Chapman and Hall.

Leonard, A. (1994) *Right from the start*, London: Scope.

Limbrick, P. (2001) *The Team Around the Child: Multi-agency service coordination for children with complex needs and their families*, Manchester: Interconnections.

Limbrick, P. (2003) *An Integrated Pathway For Assessment and Support*, Worcester: Interconnections.

McConachie, H. (1990) 'Breaking the news to family and friends: some ideas to help parents', *Mental Handicap* 19, 48–50.

McGonigal, M. J. *et al*. (1991) 'A family-centred process for the individualised family service plan', *Journal of Early Intervention* 15(1) 46–56.

Quinne, L. and Rutter, D. R. (1994) 'First diagnosis of severe mental and physical disability: A study of doctor–patient communication', *Journal of Child Psychology and Psychiatry*, 35(7) 1273–1287.

Rogers, C. R. (1980) *A Way of Being*, Boston: Houghton Mifflin.

Royal College of Nursing (1999) *Supporting parents when they are told of their child's health disorder or disability*, London: RCN.

Royal College of Psychiatrists (2004) *Psychiatric services for children and adolescents with learning disabilities*, Council Report CR123: September, London: RCP.

Russell, P. (1991) 'Working with children with physical disabilities and their families' in M. Oliver (ed.), *Social Work: Disabled People and Disabling Environments*, London: Jessica Kingsley.

Sanderson, H. (2004) 'Using Person-Centred Planning and approaches with children and families', *Learning Disability Practice*, 7(10), 16–21.

Shampan, L. (2002) *Parents have needs too! The role of counselling services for children with special needs and disabilities*, Ealing Mencap: 3Cs Counselling Service.

St John, T. (2004) 'First Impressions', *Learning Disability Practice* 7(8) October 12–14.

Warner, H. (2001) 'Children with additional needs: The transdisciplinary approach', *Paediatric Nursing* 13(6) 33–36.

6 Making contact – building relationships

Helen K. Warner

Building relationships between families and professionals

This concept will be explored within the context of an Early Intervention Nursery, considering how the principles of family centred care can be applied to both the community and acute care settings. A hierarchy of family-centred care (Hutchfield 1999) will be utilised to structure discussion (Table 6.1). This hierarchy was based on the work of Shelton and Smith-Stepanek (1995), who developed their framework of family-centred care within the context of children with learning disability.

Building relationships in the Early Intervention Unit

Parental involvement

The development of family-centred care begins when the family first attend the Early Intervention Unit. At this early stage the nurse and family meet as strangers. The role of the nurse is to establish open and honest

Table 6.1 Family-centred care

Family-centred care: Concerned with a supportive relationship based on mutual respect and trust. Parents are now expert in the needs of their child and consult professionals when in need of advice and support.

Partnership with parents: Concerned with the health care professional working with parents as a supporter and adviser to parents who are now skilled and knowledgeable in the care of their child. Shared decision making.

Parental participation: Concerned with sharing knowledge with the parents and teaching them the skills they need to care for their child and promote their development. Collaboratively relationship established.

Parental involvement: Concerned with helping the parents maintain their normal parenting role and providing the parent(s) with information and answering questions.

Source: adapted from Hutchfield (1999).

communication with the parent that enables information to be given and information requests to be addressed (Hutchfield 1999).

This dialogue provides the opportunity for the nurse to demonstrate his/her acceptance of the parents as constants in the life of their child, and as such the most important people to their child. Some parents may be wary of having the involvement of yet more professionals 'telling them what to do', and may come with unrealistic expectations that cannot be met. The challenge for the staff is to work with the parent without destroying their hopes for their child, by accepting their perspective (Nugent and Halborsen 1995) and working together on those aspects of the child's care that are not contentious. The family will need to be aware that as the child will be cared for within a multi-professional team, information will be shared on a 'need to know' basis only. In this way mutual trust and respect can be established and maintained, so that with time the more difficult areas where disagreement may exist can be explored and agreement reached that is mutually acceptable. However, this would only be the case if the care issue under debate is not one that places the child's health or safety at risk. If the child's well-being is at risk it is defensible to break parental confidentiality and in these situations the professionals may be forced to take unilateral action (NMC 2002).

The initial assessment provides the opportunity for the nurse to demonstrate his/her respect for the family's values and acknowledge their feelings even when incompatible with the listeners own beliefs and experience (Fine and Glasser 1996). Negotiating ground rules (e.g. agreeing to bring the child regularly to the unit, and not bringing the child in when they are ill) and making it clear what rights and responsibilities the family has, helps to ensure the integrity of the relationship (Bond 2001).

At this time the parents may share the role of advocate for the child. The parents maintain overall responsibility for their child, but in their absence the nurse assumes the guardianship role, and will ensure that the child's therapy is appropriately timed to fit into the child's normal activities e.g. normal eating and rest patterns. In order for the nurse to be able to assume the guardianship role, there must be a relationship underpinned by trust. However, trust does not just happen but grows and develops over time.

The development of trust

Under normal circumstances, individuals grow to know and trust each other by spending time together exchanging favours, help and confidences (Fong and Cox 1989). In this relationship, however, the amount of time and range of activities are not always available or appropriate. Families will therefore need to see observable instances of trustworthiness and will 'test' the nurse in various ways. The most common of these is to request information or to put themselves down by voicing feelings of inadequacy in their parenting skills when they find themselves unable to completely meet their child's needs unaided. Thus they may need to be reassured and reminded that they have other demands on their time, whereas the Nursery staff can be totally focused on the child, for the relatively short time the child is in their care. It is therefore essential to build a trusting relationship in order to both improve care and help to reduce parental stress and anxiety (NMC 2002).

Parental participation

Once a rapport has been established between the family and professional the relationship moves into the parental participation and partnership with parent's element of the hierarchy. Within these areas the nurse's role changes to one of teacher of the parents/carers and sharer in the care of the child. The nurse may also act as a gatekeeper at this stage (Hutchfield 1999). The parents may be faced with many challenges that could overwhelm them, and the nurse will prioritise these and help the parents to focus their energies on the things that they feel willing and able to change. Once the parents begin to see some small successes it encourages them to tackle the more difficult issues. This in a way reflects a paternalistic approach (Gillon1986) with the professional taking the lead in decision making; however, to do otherwise would place the full burden on parents and families at a time when they may not be ready to take this on.

The focus at this stage is on the sharing of knowledge with the family and reinforcing the importance of the parent's role in the continuing progress or maintenance of their child. The involvement of the multi-professional team will mean the parents have much new and often complicated information to make sense of and to put into practice. This may all be at a time when the child's sleep pattern is erratic and disturbing the sleep of the whole family (Durand 1998) so that they may be physically exhausted.

Partnership with parents

As parents become more experienced and knowledgeable they are able to become equal partners with the health professionals in the decision-making process. This partnership may not mean equal power in this context, but reflect people working together towards a common goal (Tunnard and Ryan 1991). The role of the health professional may have moved from the teacher to the supporter and advisor, which is far less directive than the teaching relationship.

To maintain the relationship it will be important for the nurse to acknowledge that the child may not be the only concern of the family. The needs of other family members, financial concerns, and employment and/or marital worries may sometimes have to take priority. The demands on parents who are caring for their child with learning disabilities are well documented, and the mismatch between the help families have and what is needed from outside agencies is also acknowledged. Mencap (2002) identified that 48 per cent of families received no support at all from outside the family, and that 80 per cent of services from professionals were poorly coordinated. However, although the involvement of service users is a central theme of recent health agendas, evidence suggests that this type of involvement is problematic and often tokenistic (Barr 1996). This would seem to suggest that it is extremely important to seek out the views of families so that the care their child receives can be improved in the light of what they believe will work for them, rather than the 'professionals' presuming to know what is best.

Family-centred care

The role of the nurse in the final stage of family-centred care includes that of counsellor and consultant. In this role the professional is in the position to support the family with practical advice as well as being a trusted listener, and the parents are respected and valued for the knowledge and skills they have acquired in order to support their child.

The specialist Health Visitor has a central role to play in the development of networks and support groups that can provide families with much valuable support and friendship.

Parents as experts

In the acute setting it is the family who are the experts regarding their own child's condition and daily care needs. This must be acknowledged and respected so that working together and sharing expertise becomes the norm. It can take a long time to establish a relationship with the child with special needs and it is very easy to make assumptions about them and their care. Nurses must be willing to learn from parents, and accept that the helping process is a two-way process. If anyone can teach us about effort and commitment it is the families of children with complex health needs. Good practice requires a combination of professional competence, good relationships with clients and colleagues and a commitment to and observance of professional ethics (Bond 2001).

Barriers to family-centred care

Although family-centred care is considered central to the care of hospitalised children, there are many barriers to providing it for children with disabilities (Robinson 1987; Darbyshire and Morrison 1995). Children's nurses have spoken about the formation of special relationships which cause nurses to cross over boundaries and sometimes be more involved than with a 'routine admission' (Ford and Turner 2001). However, as Robinson (1987) reminds us, health professionals in the acute setting are orientated to providing acute care, and the settings themselves are rarely designed to meet the special needs of children with disabilities and chronic illness.

While nurses have spoken of 'sharing the burden' and 'feeling privileged' when sharing special moments with families (Ford and Turner 2001), they have also revealed feelings of frustration and guilt when unable to provide holistic care. The more immediate needs of acutely ill children often take priority when time is limited. Minimising the long-term problems becomes a low priority. It has been suggested that true family empowerment can only occur if models of care move away from one that is medically orientated, and that junior staff have difficulties achieving partnerships due to their inexperience in using negotiating skills and their inability to deal with conflict (Valentine 1998). More experienced staff need to ensure that their junior staff have further training in interpersonal skills, communication and managing conflict.

In the acute setting it has been suggested that families need to know and trust the professionals as friends (Darbyshire and Morrison 1995). However, as Lindon and Lindon (2000) point out, although effective helping needs to be friendly, families must be treated professionally, which means with equality. Any problems that arise in forming an appropriately courteous relationship need dealing with so that they are not allowed to influence the amount or quality of help provided.

Over-involvement with children and families, without considering the opinions, knowledge and skills of multi-disciplinary team members, may lead to a lack of objectivity. Benner and Wrubel (1989) indicate that it is an art to know what nurses can offer without becoming over-involved, implying that while the experienced nurse may have developed this art, students may not yet have done so. Students may therefore require close supervision to ensure that they do not become too involved with a family, but equally need to be encouraged to be adequately involved in order to be helpful to the family as well as for their own learning and self-growth.

Active listening

The importance of listening lies in enabling the families to feel understood. Good listening is much more complex than it may at first seem, involving an awareness of the verbal and non-verbal cues of the other person. Listening is an active process, which also involves observing and reading the emotion behind the verbal message, noting any conflict which may need challenging (Egan 1998). The listener also listens to his/her own feelings which may be aroused and which may interfere with the helping process if not effectively dealt with elsewhere, e.g. in clinical supervision. When helpers understand and can control their own reactions, they are much more capable of receiving loud and clear signals from their clients (Kennedy and Charles 1992).

It is also necessary to be able to respond to the speaker, communicating that the spoken message has been received accurately enabling the client to feel understood (Egan 1998). Responses made by the nurse require sensitivity and a sense of timing which builds on what seems natural and appropriate (Kennedy and Charles 1992), and care needs to be taken when choosing words of response in order not to appear to blame or placate. Thus a great deal of effort has to be put into listening, totally focusing on the speaker without losing the thread of what is being said. This kind of listening can be quite draining and it is therefore important for the listener to have a good support system so that when listening, he/she does not become overloaded and therefore ineffective. Meeting with colleagues or having regular clinical supervision is a way of helping to keep things in perspective and enables some of the stress related to the use of these skills to be diffused.

In the acute setting

Families may be feeling vulnerable and anxious, or even angry that their child needs a hospital admission. Demonstrating respect for and acceptance of how they are feeling is the first step to developing family-centred care and of gaining the family's trust. Parents need to feel safe and have confidence in the organisation to support them. The professional who is trustworthy, demonstrating integrity and maturity, and who has high standards of care will be able to develop a trusting relationship with them in accordance with the NMC (2002).

Lifelong users of children's services

Children with complex disabilities and long-term needs are likely to have repeated hospital admissions, with all the difficulties any other child experiences when hospitalised, but hugely magnified (Warner 2000). It is vital to understand that there is already a multi-professional team around the child, so that colleagues within the team are deserving of the same respectful participative approaches as the families (Darbyshire and Morrison 1995). As the NMC (2002) states, 'good care should be the product of a good team', which means cooperation and collaboration of all the health, social and education team members around the child, both for the duration of the admission and when planning to discharge the child. Children's nurses are in a good position to coordinate the care of these special children and ensure appropriate colleagues are involved as necessary e.g. the child's physiotherapist, occupational therapist and speech and language therapist rather than the hospital on-call therapists who will not be familiar with the child.

Contracts and boundary-setting

If it is made clear from the start what families may expect from the service and what is expected from them they will be enabled to feel more confident and in control of their lives. To negotiate who will do what and when with regard to daily living activities and nursing care, will help to enable a family to take appropriate breaks without feeling that if they are not present, their child's needs will not be met. It will also help families to have more realistic expectations of the staff and vice versa. Nurses, perhaps, need to be more proactive in ensuring that these ground rules are in place, which will promote trust and confidence in the staff as long as they are adhered to. Any changes must be discussed and agreed with the family and as the partnership develops professionals and family again work together towards a common goal (Tunnard and Ryan 1991). In this way the families can be empowered with sufficient information to be able to make informed decisions and influence their child's care.

Consistency of care-giving

King, King and Rosenbaum (1996) found that continuity of care is an important aspect of care and that information exchange, support, respect and being involved as a partner in care is important irrespective of socio-economic background. They concluded that taking a family-centred approach to care influences client satisfaction and adherence to recommendations as it meets the basic human need for 'control, respect and support'. However children with special needs, chronic illness and long-term needs are likely to have repeated hospital admissions and there may be a high turnover of staff. If the same people are not available on subsequent admissions, senior staff can ensure consistency of care by completing a summary, which can be updated on each admission and kept at the front of the child's medical notes. Alternatively, or in addition to this, the child may have a personal profile (Tippett 2001; Stanislawski 1997) containing all the information necessary to meet his/her daily care requirements. These measures will ensure that new staff and students can quickly familiarise themselves with the individual child's most recent care without the family feeling they have to repeat their 'story' each time.

Self-awareness

The importance of active listening has already been explored. Actively listening requires single-minded concentration and the ability to set aside one's own preoccupations in order to become wholly available to the other person (Hough 1996). Anyone in a helping relationship should think about furthering his/her own self-development and self-awareness in order to provide a high quality service.

Although an often difficult and painful process it is essential to understand oneself more fully. If health professionals are not in touch with their own feelings they will be unable to understand the wide range of feelings experienced by parents in the acute setting, and may even confuse their own feelings with those of the parent.

There is also often a risk that the health professional gets drawn into behaviour that is a reaction to the behaviour of the parent. Parents and helper may then get caught up into an emotional 'battle'. This emotional experience can be called a 'reactive process' and we have all had some experience of situations like this; although the content of such situations may differ, the emotional process that occurs remains the same. Another model of understanding the reactive process is the Drama Triangle, which originates in Transactional Analytic thinking (Karpman 1968). The Drama Triangle suggests that when we are caught up in reactive processes we interact with each other from three possible stances; 'Rescuer', 'Victim' or 'Persecutor'. In practice, once caught up in the process it is easy to become ensnared and to oscillate between two of the stances in the relationship between ourselves and another.

The Drama Triangle

RESCUER

'I can help you, I know what is best for you.'

VICTIM	PERSECUTOR
'Leave me alone. I can't help it.'	'After all I have done, and you still don't change.'

The consequence of becoming stuck in reactive processes can be that most of the energy goes into the reactive process, leaving little energy to focus on the need for change, and the focus of all the adults concerned is taken away from the child. Thus clear communication and partnership can become almost impossible to achieve. It is therefore important to recognise when a relationship is caught into a reactive process, and to develop skills in helping the process of communication to move back towards a balance. An awareness of how we react in different situations is essential to the creation of effective nurse–client relationships particularly where the nurse uses him/her 'self' as therapy, that is *being* something to help the client rather than *doing* something to help (Carpenter et al. 1996).

This is particularly important in Child Protection work where emotional content is high for all concerned and it is therefore extremely likely that professionals will get caught up in reactive processes at some point in their work. Smith (1992) asserted that nurses cannot be blamed for fearing having to deal with a patient who is struggling with violent emotions. However, Egan (1998) argues that it is important when working with any kind of reluctance and resistance to suggested changes that, rather than reacting to it, being inventive in finding ways to work with the resistance and accepting that this is how they are feeling, is the most effective way of helping. Also, as Rogers (1961) suggested, adopting a person-centred approach, which involves 'warm positive regard' and 'empathy, respect and congruence' towards family members, supporting them to use their own strengths to cope, will help nurses to remain positive.

Identifying and understanding personal prejudices and blind spots is another aspect of self-awareness, and can be a difficult area to address since most of us tend to ignore our shortcomings. However, without an acknowledgement of these prejudices, true humility and unpretentiousness are impossible and there is a danger that self-importance will flaw the relationship with clients (Hough 1996). The process of self-awareness enables the carer to learn to identify and separate their own issues and problems from those of other people. These issues may then be dealt with, leaving the carer more 'available' i.e. mentally and physically present for the client's needs, and not for their own.

Clinical supervision

Tyler and Cushway (1992) argue that constantly dealing with the pain of others will inevitably take its toll. Lokk and Arnetz (1997) demonstrated that with emotional and psychological support the stress levels and sick leave of staff may be reduced. In an ideal world all nurses would have access to clinical supervision, which would provide the necessary support to enable them to keep things in perspective and remain objective.

Clinical supervision has been slow to be recognised as useful for nurses outside such specialties as mental health and counselling. However, it is essential for the user of counselling skills. It is defined as regular and formal non-managerial supervision, which is primarily concerned with the well-being of the client and secondarily with that of the practitioner (BAC 1999). It is difficult to remain objective when as personally involved in a relationship as the use of counselling skills demands, since working with the distress and difficulties of others can affect the helper (Bond 2001). Thus, supervision can provide support to recognise and manage the emotional impact of using counselling skills in order to enhance effectiveness and to prevent burnout so that the needs of the client can be focused on exclusively (NMC 2002). It is also a way to protect client confidentiality so that a user of counselling skills does not inadvertently disclose information inappropriately when seeking personal support.

Clinical supervision is therefore not a luxury but an essential part of support for nurses. Supervision is also a way of helping the professional to develop both personally and professionally so that the family is protected from any potential blind-spots the professional may have in his/her own awareness and attitudes, thus ensuring standards of care. Hawkins and Shohet (1992) observed that a good supervisory relationship is the best way to ensure that we remain open to ourselves and to our clients. It is a process designed to develop the professional's own 'inner supervisor'. Developing a healthy internal supervisor allows reflection to take place while the professional is working and has been defined as being autonomous, and helping the helper to respond appropriately to the immediacy of the present moment.

In conclusion

There is clearly not the same amount of time in the acute setting as in the early intervention nursery for forming relationships and building trust. In the early intervention nursery, trust is established through first working with parents, winning their trust before the trust of their children. What may make them feel safe, such as a very few consistent care-givers and a routine that with time becomes familiar, may not be available or possible in hospital and there may also be unpleasant procedures that have to be carried out.

In the acute setting it may be difficult for a child to be trusting, if their parent is not present. It may also be difficult for the parents, who may feel very protective of their child when confronted with nurses who may not be familiar with their child's condition and daily care routine, but nevertheless need their help with the current episode of illness or surgery, and nursing care required. The situation may also be difficult for nurses who may recognise their own lack of knowledge, perceive the family as experts and somehow need to develop a relationship so that the parents will be able to trust them.

Implications for nurses

There is much that nurses can do. Nurses can acknowledge the expertise of parents and learn from it, so that they may demonstrate their ability to meet the daily care requirements of individual children with disabilities. Nurses perhaps also need to explain to parents that sometimes care has to be prioritised. However, if the daily care is appropriately negotiated, in a realistic way, and adhered to, the child's needs should be met. There is an implication for staffing levels since the child with disabilities will need more time than other children to ensure that his/her needs are adequately met especially if we are to minimise the effects of hospitalisation. Casey (2001:3) summed it up in six words: 'Enough staff with the right skills'. Having enough staff with the right skills would ensure that high-quality evidence-based care would be achieved and that communication with children and families would also be well managed. Play specialists may have an important part to play in ensuring that the child with disabilities is stimulated and his/her developmental needs are catered for.

Other things nurses can do:

- Acknowledge their own learning deficits.
- Become more self-aware and learn to be assertive, which will enable the other person's rights to be respected as well as their own.
- Become more effective users of interpersonal skills and learn to recognise when they are caught up in reactive processes, discussing it with others e.g. in supervision.
- Anticipate the reactive process and resistance and negotiate work with parents so that it is clear who is doing what and when.

- Reflect on their own assumptions about families and become aware of the impact on their work.
- Ensure that they have a good support system in place e.g. clinical supervision or for the student, a mentor and peer support.
- Acknowledge the diversity of response to the diagnosis of disability.
- Reduce the number of times the same questions are asked of a family by keeping an up to date summary at the front of the child's notes.
- Use communication passports or personal profiles (Stanislawski 1997; Tippett 2001), which will aid in the understanding of the child's perspective.

Nothing can be accomplished without a trusting relationship between nurses and the families of children with disabilities, first being established. Only when we have their trust can we begin to meet, more fully, the needs of the children and families entrusted to our care. Above all we need to remember that nursing goals should be 'complementary to the child's overall multi-disciplinary intervention programme' (Hooton 1995, p. 167).

References

Barr, O. (1996) 'Developing Services for people with learning disabilities which actively involve family members: a review of the literature', *Health and Social Care in the Community*, 4(2): 103–112.

Benner, P. and Wrubel, J. (1989) *The Primacy of Caring*, Menlo Park: Addison Wesley.

Beresford, P., Croft, S., Evans, C. and Harding, T. (2000) 'Quality in Personal Social Services: The Developing Role of User group involvement in the UK' chapter 19 in C. Davies, L. Finlay and A. Bullman (eds) *Changing practice in Health and Social Care*, London: The Open University and Sage Publications.

Bond, T. (2001) 'British Association of Counselling and Psychotherapy's new Ethical Framework – An introduction', *Healthcare Counselling and Psychotherapy Journal*, Oct. (1, 2) 21–22.

British Association for Counselling (1999) *Code of Ethics and Practice*, Rugby: BAC.

Carpenter, D., Turnbull J. and Kay, A. (1996) *Mental Health and Learning Disability*, London: Macmillan Magazines Ltd.

Casey, A. (2001) (Editorial) 'Six Words Say It All' *Paediatric Nursing* 13(7) Sept. 3.

Darbyshire, P. and Morrison, H. (1995) 'Empowering parents of children with special needs', *Nursing Times*, 91(32) 26–28.

Durand, V. M. (1998) *Sleep Better – A Guide to Improving sleep for children with Special needs*, London: Paul Brookes.

Egan, G. (1998) *The Skilled Helper* (6th edn.) London: Brookes/Cole, ITP.

Fine, S. and Glasser, P. (1996) *The First Helping Interview*, London: Sage.

Fong, M. and Cox, B. (1989) 'Trust as an underlying dynamic in the counselling process' chapter 3 in W. Dryden (ed.) *Key Issues for Counselling in Action*, London: Sage.

Ford, K. and Turner, de S. (2001) 'Stories seldom told: paediatric nurses' experiences of caring for hospitalised children with special needs, and their families', *Journal of Advanced Nursing*, 33(3) 228–295.

Gillon, R. (1986) *Philosophical Medical Ethics*, Chichester: John Wiley.

Hawkins, P. and Shohet, R. (1992) *Supervision in the Helping Professions*, Milton Keynes: Open University Press.

Hooton, S. (1995) 'Learning disabilities, children and their families', in B. Carter and A. Dearmun (eds) *Child Health Care Nursing*, Oxford: Blackwell Science.

Hough, M. (1996) *Counselling Skills*, Harlow: A.W. Longman.

Hutchfield, K. (1999) 'Family-centred care: a concept analysis' *Journal of Advanced Nursing* 29(5) 1178–1187.

Hutchfield, K. and Parsons, M. (2003) 'Working with Regular Users of Children's Services Groups – an Educational Experience', *Paediatric Nursing* 15(2) 36–38.

Karpman, S. (1968) 'Fairy Tales and Script Drama Analysis', *Transactional Analysis Bulletin* 7, 39–43.

Kennedy, E. and Charles, S. (1992) *On Becoming a Counsellor*, Dublin: Gill and Macmillan.

King, G., King, S. M. and Rosenbaum, P. (1996) 'Interpersonal aspects of care giving and Client Outcomes' *Ambulatory Child Health*, 2,151–160.

Lindon, J. and Lindon, L. (2000) *Mastering Counselling Skills*, London: Macmillan.

Lokk, J. and Arnetz, B. (1997) 'Psychophysiological concomitants of an organisational change in healthcare personnel: Effects of a controlled intervention study', *Psychotherapy and Psychosomatics*, 66(2) 74–77.

Mencap (2002) *No Ordinary Life: The support needs of families caring for children and adults with profound and multiple learning disabilities*, London: Mencap.

Nugent, W. and Halborsen, H. (1995) 'Testing the effects of active listening', *Research on Social Work Practice*, 5(2) 152–175.

Nursing and Midwifery Council (2002) *Code of Professional Conduct*, NMC.

Rees, S. (1998) *A Parent's Experience of Hospital Admission*, RCN Children with Disabilities SIG Annual Conference, Dec. 12th.

Robinson, C. (1987) 'Roadblocks to family-centred care when a chronically ill child is Hospitalised', *Maternal Child Nursing*, 16, 181–193.

Rogers, C. (1961) *On Becoming a Person*, London: Constable.

Shelton, T. and Smith-Stepanek, J. (1995) 'Excerpts from family-centred care for children needing specialised health and development services', *Paediatric Nursing* 21(4) 362–364.

Smith, P. (1992) *The Emotional Labour of Nursing*, London: Macmillan.

Stanislawski, N. (1997) 'Lorna's Book', *Talking Sense*, Summer, 26–27.

Tippett, A. (2001) 'All About Me: Documentation for children with special needs', *Paediatric Nursing* 13(10) Dec., 34–35.

Tunnard, J., and Ryan, M. (1991) 'What does the Children Act mean for family members?' *Children and Society*: 5, 67–75.

Tyler, P. A. and Cushway, D. (1992) 'Stress, Coping and Mental Well-being in Hospital Nurses', *Stress Medicine* 8, 91–98.

Valentine, F. (1998) 'Empowerment: Family-Centred Care', *Paediatric Nursing* 10(1) Feb. 24–7.

Warner, H. K. (2000) 'Making the Invisible, Visible' *Journal of Child Health Care* 4(3) Autumn, 123–126.

7 Movement, learning and having fun

Helen K. Warner

In the past, children who were mentally and physically challenged often became self-fulfilling prophecies of 'they'll never be able to do anything' (Nus 2001). Now that attitudes have changed, as much independence as possible is encouraged through early intervention, and society is increasingly supportive of people with additional needs, to enable them to lead productive and satisfying lives.

Most of us take for granted the ability to move, to walk across a room, sit in a chair or simply to sit still. Children without disabilities become able to sit unsupported, walk, talk, and to actively play and participate in events in their environment without undue effort. They learn from 'doing' and through play, children under age 3 years being unwilling to accept being trained or taught (Nielsen 1997). For children with multiple disabilities, however, it may be frustratingly difficult to achieve any of the normal milestones. Thus it becomes necessary to actively provide opportunities to enable these children to 'do' and to learn. Nielsen (1997) suggests that learning at the developmentally appropriate age is more beneficial for children than (chronological) age-appropriate education or training, since the traditional methods of teaching and training have failed to facilitate development in many instances. The development of infants and children occurs simultaneously in several areas, each area influencing their abilities in the others.

This chapter will discuss the early development of movement, knowledge of which is crucial when attempting to enable the child with disabilities to learn how to play and therefore learn about the world around him/her. The aim is to enable the reader to have an understanding of how the skills of movement and play normally evolve and some of the difficulties that children with disabilities may experience if this process is interrupted for any reason. There will be a discussion regarding sensory integration and finally some suggestions as to what may be done in the acute setting to minimise the child's physical regression as a result of hospitalisation.

Learning to move

Since infants and young children learn by 'doing' it seems clear that they first need to be able to move and be enabled to master the multitude of skills necessary for independent daily living. Movement begins in utero from three to four months following conception. The foetus begins moving his arms, legs and mouth. As he grows, the space available becomes smaller so that, as he stretches out his arms and legs, he can feel the uterine walls. Thus he is learning to tighten his muscles as he bends and stretches, also learning that movements have consequences i.e. if he puts his hand to his mouth he is able to suck his hand.

After birth, the flexed position of the newborn gradually changes to a position of extension (Hall and Hill 1996). The infant now learns that when he moves his arms and legs there is a new tactile experience, and instead of feeling the uterine walls he can feel the cot sheets or side of the cot, his parents or the air around him. This sensory-motor stage, described by Piaget (1975) is the stage of 'feeling' rather than thinking. Although initially unintentional, the infant without disabilities has no difficulty in learning to move intentionally. The infant learns by receiving tactile (touch), visual, auditory and olfactory feedback from the movements he makes, interpreting and integrating them in his brain. It is the constant interpretation and adjustment to new information, which encourages his further exploration, and which enables him to learn. He keeps himself stimulated by kicking, sucking his hand, bending and stretching his fingers and by babbling. Sensory information is also provided from additional sources (Table 7.1).

Following on from these basic senses, sensory-motor skills emerge. In the newborn, initial postures, and movements of limbs are dominated by primary reflexes (Hall and Hill 1996). These gradually disappear as increasing control of neck and shoulder muscles is achieved. Table 7.2 shows the early developmental milestones of movement.

Posture and movement development depends on tone and reciprocal innervation (Hall and Hill 1996). Postural tone is the ability to hold the body upright against gravity, while being ready to move and reciprocal innervation is what happens when one set of muscles contract and the opposite set of muscles relax. Also essential for normal motor function are the righting reactions and equilibrium reactions, which are automatic postural reactions to protect the child from falling. Thus between five to seven months it is

Table 7.1 Sources of sensory information

---

1. *Proprioception* (the sense of a joint's position in space).
2. *The Vestibular sense* (the ability to interpret movement in relation to the earth's surface, upright, upside down, lying sideways).
3. *The Kinaesthetic sense* (conscious perception of movement, weight, resistance and position of a body part).

Source: adapted from Cantu (2002).

Table 7.2 Early developmental milestones of movement

0–3 months	the infant gains head control
3–4 months	examines hands and fingers with hands together in the midline
4 months	the infant begins to support himself on his arms in prone position and can pick up objects; holds two objects simultaneously and begins to transfer from hand to hand
5 months	bridging – the infant lifts his bottom up when supine
5–6 months	begins to rotate and roll, reaching out for toys
7 months	beginnings of fine motor development
8–12 months	sits unsupported, crawls, creeps, pulls up to stand and cruises.

possible to see the parachute reflex in which the arms, hands and fingers extend to break a fall, and the sideways and forwards saving reflexes which make independent sitting possible.

Figure 7.1 shows how the child with normal tone and movement patterns learns to move, initially accidentally and gradually more purposefully, experiencing pleasure and success from his movements. This leads to the constant repetition and practice of an increasing variety of movements, which as the child continues to experience success, increases his motivation until he achieves a skill. Once achieved, the skill itself provides sensory feedback to the brain, which in turn reinforces the normal tone. Thus constant repetition is vital, for the movement to become included in the child's 'automatic' repertoire.

Infants also use movement as a means to express themselves, and they gradually use more movements for communication, as well as a response to games initiated by an adult (Nielsen 1997).

In the early years, initiating fine movements of one limb will cause the opposite limb to move in a similar way (Hall and Hill 1996). Associated movements such as tongue protrusion and facial grimacing will also occur when motor skills are performed. As the child develops and matures movement becomes more precise, and the associated movements diminish although they may sometimes still be observed in the adult who is challenging their fine motor skills e.g. threading a needle. Hand skills also continue to mature throughout childhood, with increasing control over finger/thumb movements.

Learning to play

A great deal has been written about the importance of play in enhancing children's development in all areas, physical, cognitive, social, emotional and spiritual. Development of these areas is interdependent, and play skills also develop alongside the physical, cognitive and motor abilities that support their emergence (Mailloux and Burke 1997). Early play is influenced by the drive for sensory-motor experiences and infants spend a great deal of time in exploratory play, both seeking and experiencing tactile, vestibular,

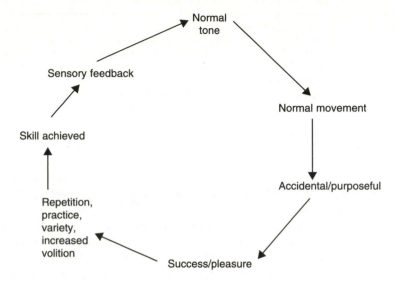

Figure 7.1 Acquisition of normal movement patterns.

proprioceptive, visual and auditory input, looking for new challenges as well as familiar and comforting sensory experiences. As the infant develops voluntary, controlled movements so his play becomes more constructive and he begins to have ideas of what to do and to plan how to do it.

During the pre-school years imaginary and social play skills emerge and include the use of language and symbolic play. As children play constructively the sensory and motor aspects of their play allow more complex conceptual and social functions to emerge e.g. balance, hand–eye coordination and the coordinated use of the hands as when riding a bicycle or playing a musical instrument. At this stage the child is learning to maintain a calm and alert state, develop new skills and learning about interacting and relating to others.

The school years bring play in which rules and skills become more important. An intact nervous system that ensures efficient sensory integration is necessary to allow a child to enjoy activities that are highly dependent on these functions and which also affect the child's social status, motivation and self-esteem. This is of particular significance as self-consciousness and peer evaluation of the child's performance become increasingly important (Mailloux and Burke 1997). As children move into adolescence, team participation in organised games and sports and special interest groups for activities such as music, dancing, and discussion become more significant and their leisure may be used to develop craftsmanship, special talents and hobbies.

At all stages of development, the importance of laughter and fun must not be forgotten. Fun and laughter fertilise the brain and also the inner spirit, and help us both to respect the way we feel and also how other people feel. We are pre-programmed to laugh with others, and there are areas in the brain that can be stimulated to cause laughter (BBC2 1998), both tickling and laughter helping to develop play. As we begin to realise the importance of play and its function in enabling children to focus their attention, it may be that children who find playing difficult e.g. children with ADHD, need to be perceived as different rather than disruptive, so that they do not feel blamed for their anti-social behaviour which may result in poor self-esteem.

Unfortunately opportunities to play are generally declining due to the dangers of playing in the street, and in schools due to the pressure to spend more time in lessons. However the importance of play must not be minimised and more time in the classroom has been shown, not to produce more academic ability, but to produce more inattention (BBC2 1998). Children with ADHD, for example, were shown to have smaller frontal lobes and be more playful. The more play they have as children, it has been suggested, the less impulsive they are as adults. A programme at the University of California uses therapeutic play with some success, whereby if the children are disruptive, they are encouraged to be even more stimulated and excited and given praise for their self-control and eye contact rather than criticised for fidgeting (BBC2 1998). However, this is an expensive and demanding programme and some children still require the support of Ritalin.

Sensory integration

Thirty years ago, Ayres (1979) described sensory integration as the organisation of sensory information applied to daily activities, which in the case of children, is play. Thus if there is a problem with the integration of the sensory messages received by the brain, there will be a disruption in the child's ability to play and interact with others which will be demonstrated by his behaviour. Examples of sensory integration dysfunction that can severely limit play in young children are tactile defensiveness, auditory defensiveness and gravitational insecurity (Mailloux and Burke 1997). Children may be highly sensitive (hyper-reactive), or unresponsive (hypo-reactive) to their environment.

Tactile defensiveness

The child's avoidance of tactile exploration through hand and mouth manipulation of objects will limit his range of experiences and therefore the skills he develops. The infant who avoids putting objects in his mouth will have difficulty accepting solid food, forming words and handling toys. This in turn will affect his visual and manipulative skills.

At the pre-school stage of development this same child will find sand, water, finger paints and play-dough etc. aversive, and as social play emerges alongside other children, the accidental bumping into each other when sharing play materials may cause a negative reaction in the child. The tactile defensiveness may cause him to squirm, pull or run away and cry or shut down completely and refuse to participate as a way of protecting himself from sensory overload (Mailloux and Burke 1997).

Auditory defensiveness

Similarly the child with auditory defensiveness may be over-sensitive to sound, so that sounds that are meant to be encouraging, rewarding or comforting are perceived as irritating, or even frightening and will cause the child to withdraw from play. In the long term this may have consequences on his social, physical and cognitive skills (Mailloux and Burke 1997).

Gravitational insecurity

Another example of sensory integration dysfunction is the child with gravitational insecurity who was described by Ayres (1979) as a child who feels irrational fear and distress in relation to movement and change of position. As infants they may be swung or rocked less, due to their negative reactions, which reduces the vestibular sensations received and so the child is at risk of having delayed development of their muscle tone, balance, equilibrium reactions and hand–eye coordination, in addition to a reduced desire to participate socially as a result of a prolonged state of fear (Mailloux and Burke 1997). Other children may have difficulty sensing where their bodies are in space and may be perceived as clumsy. They may cry, remain frozen to one spot and be unable to plan the movements necessary to move on (Cantu 2002).

When children reach school age, and their skills are becoming more refined, more subtle difficulties may become apparent. Vestibular-bilateral and sequencing disorders can severely disrupt the child's ability to perform certain skills and academic tasks which younger children would not be expected to do. Confusion about directionality (left versus right) often co-exists with bilateral integration problems which causes difficulty in knowing which way to run during e.g. a football or netball game and the child experiences embarrassment and failure (Mailloux and Burke 1997).

Other sensory integration problems, which may not become apparent until school age, were described by Ayres (1985) as developmental dyspraxia, a disorder in which there is difficulty in ideation, planning and/or the execution of unfamiliar tasks. For most adults the daily activities of living have become automatic but children are constantly learning new skills as they move towards independence. Thus if a child has difficulty in forming ideas and a plan of action, then he will probably also have difficulty in carrying out that action (Mailloux and Burke 1997).

However, if the process which is causing problems can be identified, a paediatric physiotherapist or occupational therapist can select appropriate activities to increase the child's tolerance for particular stimuli or decrease their craving for them. This can then be reinforced both at home and at school and a collaborative effort may be made toward treatment and success (Cantu 2002).

Children with disabilities

The majority of infants with disabilities are born with the same abilities to move as children without disabilities, asserts Nielsen (1997). However they may not have the same opportunities to learn, due to prematurity, a motor disability such as cerebral palsy and/or a sensory deprivation e.g. visual impairment. Intentional movements are only learnt when the child's own brain instigates the movement. Thus the infant needs to become conscious of how to perform certain movements and develop his kinaesethic sense, which cannot be learnt when an adult performs the movements for him. The infant who has difficulty moving may become passive and forget how to move if he is not provided with opportunities to experience movement successfully and to have sufficient opportunities to practise the movement.

If the infant is visually challenged he will require environmental intervention to make it meaningful for him to move (Nielsen 1997). It also seems logical that he will benefit from tactile, auditory, and olfactory experiences. Similarly the child who is unable to move due to spasticity of his muscles, and is unable to combine movements with visual experiences, will require environmental intervention to enable him to have meaningful opportunities to move. Should the child have abnormal movement patterns due to abnormal muscle tone, his movements may become stereotyped due to lack of appropriate feedback, which in turn increases the tone, ultimately leading to contractures and deformities, when the cycle recommences (Figure 7.2).

The more the child uses their muscle spasticity to help them move, the tighter the muscles become. It is therefore vital to work towards reducing the effects of the increased tone to allow the child to experience more normal movements. This may be achieved by using a variety of positions such as standing, sitting, the use of lycra suits, orthotic splinting, and above all, correct handling and positioning as advised by a paediatric physiotherapist. The child will require a considerable amount of practice before the movements become a natural part of the child's repertoire of movement. Correct positioning enhances function, provides support that can free the hands for manipulation and allows participation in activities at a variety of developmental levels, maximising access to the environment (Procter 1989). Thus, core stability allows the child's limbs to move from their base without fear of loss of his antigravity position.

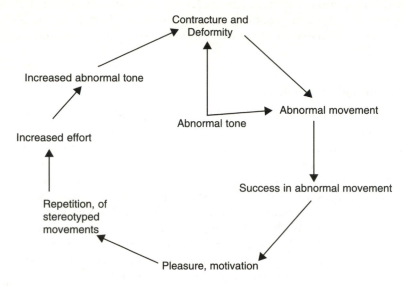

Figure 7.2 Acquisition of abnormal movement patterns.

Premature babies

Good positioning begins in the Special Care Baby Unit (SCBU), since pre-mature babies are at risk of sensory-motor developmental delay. Pre-term babies are unable to develop the physiological flexion that is vital for the development of normal movement and control, since they are seldom big enough, and will therefore have low muscle tone (hypotonia). They therefore have difficulty combating gravity to develop flexion. Poor positioning reinforces the development of abnormal patterns of movement. The typical flattening of the sides of the head of pre-term infants is due to the effects of gravity and the full weight of the brain tissue flattening the soft cartilaginous skull bones between it and the cot mattress (Turrill 1992). Infants in SCBU are restrained and attached to life support machines and are therefore unable to experience normal movement. They are subjected to frequent invasive procedures, which together with the stressful environment may contribute to negative behaviour.

Consequently rigid positioning and an inability to lie still or relax may be seen, with no pleasure to be had from being cuddled. Prolonged lying in the prone or supine position results in a frog-like posture due to excessive scapular retraction, the arms up and out away from the body, which encourages the scapulae to be pulled in towards each other. This can lead to difficulty in bringing the hands together or to the mouth, which are important steps in development. Children who are born prematurely therefore first have to learn how to be flexed before they can begin to extend purposefully. Research has shown that premature babies may become dyspraxic or clumsy and uncoordinated with no sense of space, and also have a poor attention span, all of which can lead to a delay in sitting, crawling and object manipulation (Hall and Hill 1996).

Good and careful positioning can help to reduce the developmental delay of premature babies. The provision of boundaries or walls constructed from soft towels helps the baby feel secure, and offers a firm surface to push against. Facial moulding, which can temporarily make the infant look a little odd, and is thought to have some effect on bonding, between parents and baby, may be reduced by an air- or water-filled glove placed under the infant's head to enable a feeling of security which may also lead to a reduction in ventilation requirements and less energy being expended. Thus good positioning aims to encourage the development of flexion, to avoid excessive extension and should promote symmetry to avoid iatrogenic malformations including head moulding (Turrill 1992).

In the early intervention nursery

The enriched environment provided by the nursery staff, and the therapists who support them, aims to begin to unlock the potential of children with disabilities and to lay the foundations for future learning so that ultimately they may lead productive and satisfying lives wherever possible. The nursery exists to provide a positive experience for children, some of whom may not otherwise have a positive experience at this stage due to parental grieving and coming to terms with their situation. Most parents need a break from their child at times, but the families of the children who attend may not have the support of the extended family for a variety of reasons. Thus the nursery is often the first place outside of the home where parents may leave their children for a short time, knowing that their child is actively learning.

Early Intervention

Early Intervention is not a cure for a disabling condition. However, it is underpinned by the belief that the early years of learning are critically important and can be targeted to maximise the learning potential of children by providing meaningful environmental experiences that address particular needs. Early learning forms the basis for more complex levels of performance. Simple learning skills such as sitting, holding an object, exploring and communicating are important foundations for the future acquisition of skills and competencies needed for school and adulthood.

Early Intervention also provides support, instruction and information for care-givers and families. It can help parents deal constructively with the grief and distress they may experience from having a child with disabilities or developmental delays. Practical instruction concerning ways of managing their child and maximising their child's potential is provided. Also provided is information for families about where to get further assistance such as counselling and social services and support. It is a way of supporting parents in helping their child become a more social and independent person. Without correct handling and instruction, children with disabilities or who are at risk for developmental delays may develop a variety of undesirable behaviours, which may be disruptive or secondarily disabling. Early Intervention aims to prevent or minimise the development of these behaviours.

Learning in the early intervention nursery

The three optimal requirements for learning as described by Nielsen (1997) are a receptive and alert child, according to his level of development; a quality environment that will arouse the child's interest and curiosity; and a cooperative and interested adult who makes objects available, shares the child's interest and responds to his signals and vocalisations in an appropriate way. Detailed knowledge of the sequences of early learning helps the nursery staff to provide appropriate opportunities for the children to learn, and to recognise whether a child has missed a step in his development. Collaborative working between the nursery staff and the child's therapists provides suggestions to enable the child to learn the missing steps and be able to progress in his/her development.

By adopting a therapeutic approach to the care of the children during all their activities, nursery staff maximise their learning potential. However, it is true to say that children with disabilities may need many more opportunities to practise separating objects before they become able to play constructively, than children without disabilities (Nielsen 1997). When a child has mastered transferring objects from hand to hand he will need toys that are easy to separate, and a willing adult to reconstruct the toy each time he pulls it apart, until the child indicates that he has had enough. Banging games are important from age 8 months onwards, and may be played many times daily. If a child shows no sign of wanting to bang his toys he may need to be shown how and encouraged to do so.

Banging games are followed by pouring games, and games such as emptying a toy box before learning how to fill it. These steps must be mastered before the child will be ready to play constructively. Similarly when a child is ready to play stacking games it usually begins with the adult stacking and the child knocking down the objects until the child begins to imitate the adult and attempt to stack for him/herself. It may take up to 1–2 years for the child to successfully learn to stack, with an adult facilitating the play on a daily basis (Nielsen 1997). In addition, a child with disabilities may get 'stuck' at any level of development and need active help to move on. Many children can get stuck on casting, or throwing, and may benefit from games where objects are deliberately thrown into a container. However this needs to be incorporated into everyday familiar settings with familiar objects rather than practising the skill out of context.

The child who has difficulty moving may need to have toys within reach and be helped to manipulate them until he can begin to move and reach out for himself, while simultaneously encouraging him to move. It is a constant balancing act to enable him to enjoy what he has already learnt and to keep him stimulated with new challenges.

In a similar way that adults become stiff and uncomfortable when in one position for too long, children with motor difficulties also need to regularly change position, and the nursery staff are advised by a colleague physiotherapist, as to which positions are appropriate for individual children. Supine is generally not encouraged for children who have hypertonic muscles, as it encourages extensor tone (back and neck arching), so that nothing but the ceiling can be seen by the child. However, prone and side lying are good positions to use for play, and also a good sitting position. Each position has its advantages and disadvantages and depends on the child's ability and need. Standing may be free standing against a wall, against an adult or in a frame. This is an important position for various reasons (see Table 7.3).

For more able children, positions such as high and half kneeling are good to promote hip girdle stability. Children who have difficulty moving into and out of positions, and especially if fixed into a piece of equipment, should have their position changed at least half-hourly/hourly.

There is a variety of equipment, appliances and aids that may be used e.g. special boots, gaiters, body braces, callipers, hearing aids and glasses which are much more child friendly than they used to be. Any equipment, however, must be used carefully with advice from the child's therapists, in order not to cause more harm than good.

Table 7.3 The importance of standing

- Social height.
- Appropriate work height.
- Improves postural stability and muscle strength.
- Stretches body structures which are normally and constantly in a shortened position in sitting.
- Gives experience of standing and so, for some people teaches standing.
- Puts body weight through bone and joint structures so they are subjected to the normal forces which help to determine their development.
- Aids digestion.
- Aids kidney and bladder drainage.
- Facilitates respiration, particularly lower segments of lungs which are usually squashed.
- Improves peripheral circulation.
- Aids symmetry.

In the acute setting

The writer has attempted to illustrate the complexity of learning to move and to play, and how active intervention is often necessary to enable children with disabilities to acquire the most basic skills, and to enable them to be able to move on in their development. Although a spell in the acute setting may not be the appropriate time to learn new skills, because of the unfamiliar surroundings, and perhaps pain/discomfort, it is essential to allow the child with disabilities opportunities to use the skills he already has. It is also useful to be aware that the exact moment when a child will learn a new skill cannot be dictated, so that it must not be assumed that a new skill cannot emerge during a hospital admission. As previously stated, a lack of challenges and appropriate stimulation may lead to the child not only forgetting how to move but also to have an expectation that everything will be done for him/her (Nielsen 1997). For example, it is good practice to tell the child he is going to be moved and actively gain his cooperation and awareness of change rather than simply passively moving him.

Some children's wards now employ a play specialist, who may be of invaluable help when children with disabilities are admitted to hospital. Play specialists will generally have the time to offer appropriate activities to the children, and to ensure that they are not left on their beds for long periods with nothing to do. They can also liaise with the child's therapists if there are any doubts about how to position the child for play and other activities.

Parents, too, will provide an important source of information about their child's abilities. It is vital to have knowledge of the child's usual skills and not presume on the picture presented by the child if he is acutely ill. Parents' help can also be enlisted by asking them to bring in any special seating or standing equipment the child usually uses.

Children's nurses also need to be proactive in asking the families if the child has a personal profile *and to read it before* any 'hands on' care is attempted. Children's nurses can also ensure that other health professionals in the multi-disciplinary team both see and read the child's profile.

Children's nurses can adopt a therapeutic approach to the care of these children, in the same way as the early intervention nursery staff. If they are mindful that the children are children first and always, with all the needs of any other child, as well as specific needs relating to their disability, this will ensure that children's nurses demonstrate respect, while also giving some control back to the child.

One way of helping these children maintain their skills would be to ensure that there is a sensory toy box on the ward with appropriate toys to interest and stimulate the senses. Toys need to be brightly coloured and of high interest to encourage interaction and teach cause and effect, remembering for example that yellow is a good colour for the child with poor vision, and a piece of black cloth on which to put the toys will provide a contrast and make it easier for children with poor vision to pick out the toy from the background colours, enabling them to be more focused. At the end of this chapter are some suggestions of sensory toys and where they may be obtained.

A chapter on movement and play will not be complete, however, without a reminder that play is also important to allow feelings of frustration and anger to be played out. It was Erikson (1950: 215) who stated: 'As an adult will "talk it out" following a traumatic event, to solve their tension, a child will "play it out".' Thus therapeutic play can help to alleviate stress in hospital (Doverty 1992). To be effective the child must be given complete freedom to play out his accumulated tension, frustration, insecurity, aggression, fear, bewilderment and confusion, asserts Woolfson (1990) and toys must be appropriate for the child's age and stage of development or they will quickly lose interest. The value of therapeutic play in this way cannot be overstressed in the light of the loss of autonomy that many children feel during a hospital admission. Where the child cannot play for himself, for whatever reason, it will be necessary to play for the child to enable him/her to feel understood, while also helping them to make sense of what is happening to them. In this way any potential psychological regression may also be minimised.

Children with special needs may also benefit from play preparation prior to e.g. a gastrostomy procedure. Crawford and Raven (2002) describe the use of Mickey and Minnie Mouse dolls that have gastrostomy buttons to help children to cope, understand what is going to happen to them and reduce their fear. However this kind of preparation may need to be carried out over a period of several weeks, and used in conjunction with relaxation techniques and massage, various textures and pressure to the abdomen (Crawford and Raven 2002). S. Dryden, in an unpublished report, recommends that all children are prepared for such experiences regardless of their developmental level, and that distraction techniques and play preparation are taught to families and carers.

Suggested sensory toys

Simple shape sorters and sound puzzle boxes, rainmakers, magic wands, finger paints, paper, tissue paper, ping pong balls, blowpipes (an alternative to finger painting is blow painting, a blob of paint can be placed in the centre of a large piece of paper and blown on through a straw or blowpipe to make patterns), football, candles, carnival blowers, straws, lipstick, musical instruments, simple jigsaw puzzles with large pieces which perhaps make a noise when placed correctly (good for turn taking, one piece at a time), stacking rings that also light up/play a tune, vibrating toys (good for calming some children, and which provide strong sensory feedback), a 'worry toy' such as a paper clip, rubber band or stress ball to help anxious children become calm. A 'feelie' box e.g. a shoe box with a hole cut in the top, full of different objects such as spools, plastic animals, marbles etc. and the child inserts a hand through the hole to pick out or guess what is in the box. Another useful addition to the toy box is a piece of black cloth on which to place brightly coloured toys for the visually impaired child, thus providing a contrast and making it easier to be seen.

TAC PAC or a tactile approach to communication is for children with profound learning difficulties and additional sensory impairment and for whom touch may be the primary means of contact. It contains a materials list (inexpensive household items), a CD of original music and simple instructions. A narrator introduces each simple piece of music and builds this into a story, each piece relating to a tactile activity and ending with the child wrapped in a blanket to give a feeling of safety, warmth and security. The session lasts about half an hour. It is also useful for children whose condition affects their ability to explore and play independently.

It is clear that some of these activities require close supervision so that the child does not come to any harm, due to the use of small parts which under normal circumstances a young child would not be left to play with, and this is where a play specialist's time is so invaluable. I would also urge caution with e.g. blowing out of candles and the safety aspect of having matches on the ward. However, if they are stored in a locked cupboard and only used under close supervision, they can be the source of some fun as well as encouraging the child to learn to blow and maintain this skill if already learnt. It is also important to ensure that toys are not broken and work properly so that the child does not lose interest in the cause and effect aspect of a toy, which is an important developmental stage of learning. This may mean that the sensory toys are only used under supervision and not left out for common usage. The reader will find a list of possible sources of sensory toys at the end of this chapter, but it is also important to remember that many toys can be obtained from toy markets, ordinary toyshops and even the local pet shop!

Finally it is important to remember that whatever toy or activity is offered to the child, respecting their communication as to whether they want to engage with it or not is vital, so that they are allowed to choose and have some control over what they do. In this way they will be helped to understand that what they do can have an effect on their environment, which is another aspect of cause and effect, and will help to foster their positive self esteem.

Sources of sensory toys

Vibrating snake (massage tube) can be obtained from ROMPA – Tel: 0845 2301177 for a catalogue or visit www.rompa.com

Light and Sound toys, Rainmakers and Paints can be obtained from the Early Learning Centre: Tel 08705 352352 for a catalogue or visit: www.elc.co.uk

Formative Fun is another good source for sound puzzle box: Tel: 01308 868999 or visit www.Formative-Fun.com

Vibrating toys and others can be obtained from TFH or the magic planet. Visit www.magic-planet.biz.

For Sensory Games at reasonable prices in euros that can be converted online visit www.smartazzkids.com

TAC PAC can be purchased from: *chris@shapearts.org.uk* for £15 + postage and packing and includes the CD and all the information necessary to run a TAC PAC session/or visit www.shapearts.org.uk/schools

References

Ayres, A. J. (1979) *Sensory Integration and the Child*, Los Angeles: Western Psychological Services.

Ayres, A. J. (1985) *Developmental Dyspraxia and Adult onset Apraxia*, Los Angeles: Western Psychological Services.

BBC2 (1998) *Horizon*: Television Documentary: November.

Cantu, C. O. (2002) 'Early Childhood Sensory Integration' *Exceptional Parent*, April, 47–54.

Crawford, C. and Raven, K. (2002) 'Play Preparation for children with special needs', *Paediatric Nursing*, 14(8) 27–29.

Doverty, N. (1992) 'Therapeutic use of play in hospital', *British Journal of Nursing*, 1(2) 77–80.

Erikson, E. (1950) *Childhood and Society*: Harmondsworth: Penguin.

Hall, D. M. B. and Hill, P. D. (1996) *The Child with a Disability*, Oxford: Blackwell Science Ltd.

Mailloux, Z. and Burke, J. P. (1997) 'Play and the Sensory Integrative Approach', in L. D. Parham and L. S. Fazio (eds) *Play in Occupational Therapy for Children*, Missouri, USA: Mosby.

Nielsen, L. (1997) *Early Learning Step by Step: Children with vision impairment and Multiple disabilities*, Denmark: Sikon.

Nus, S. E. (2001) 'Attitude is Everything – A Parent's perspective', *Exceptional Parent*, December, 65–67.

Piaget, J. (1975) *The Construction of Reality in the Child*, New York: Ballantine Books.

Procter, S. (1989) 'Adaptations for Independent Living', in P. Pratt and A. Allen (eds) *Occupational Therapy for Children*, Missouri, USA: Mosby.

Turrill, S. (1992) 'Supported Positioning in Intensive Care' *Paediatric Nursing*, May, 24–25.

Woolfson, R. (1990) 'Using Play as Therapy' *Nursery World*, Play Series part 2, June 14, 16–17.

Further reading

Finnie, N. R. (1997) *Handling the Young Child with Cerebral Palsy at Home* (3rd edn) Butterworth/Heinemann: Oxford.

Lear, R. (1993) *Play Helps: Toys and Activities for Children with Special Needs*, London: Heinemann.

Woolfson, R. (1990) 'Play for Children with Special Needs: Play Series Part 5', *Nursery World* July 5th, 20–21.

8 Meeting nutritional needs – more than just assistance to eat and drink

Helen K. Warner

When considering how to meet the nutritional needs of the child with disabilities, it is vital to understand the complexity of the normal development of eating and drinking patterns. Other considerations include, why we eat and the choices we make around mealtimes; the importance of the child's position and what special equipment may help to increase the child's independence. Some knowledge of the development of behavioural problems is also desirable as past experiences may influence the sensation of swallowing e.g. tube feeding or nasopharyngeal suctioning. From the above it is already clear that meeting the needs of children with disabilities is complex, and the most effective approach to working is multi-disciplinary, family-centred care (Carpenter 1997). It also follows that the roles of the 'feeding' team also need to be considered.

The reason disabled children develop feeding problems is linked to their early development, for example their muscle tone influencing their oral structures. This chapter will discuss the above considerations and attempt to offer some insight into the complex process of eating and drinking so that the professional carer, whether in hospital, respite settings or schools, may confidently assist their clients to enjoy mealtimes without disempowering them. Hopefully, reading this chapter will also help to reduce the loss of independence that so often occurs when carers do not fully appreciate the time and preparation that is necessary to facilitate the child with disability's learning to eat independently (Warner 2000).

In order to ingest food orally, the efficiency of the child's swallow reflex may need assessing by the speech therapist, radiologist and paediatrician, who all have an important role to play in this assessment. An absent or poor swallow reflex places the infant/child at risk of choking or developing aspiration pneumonia. Therefore, if the swallow reflex is not adequate for the child to safely receive nutrition orally, alternative means of meeting the child's nutritional needs must be used. These commonly include feeding via a naso-gastric tube or gastrostomy.

The importance of developing eating and drinking skills

Mealtimes provide the opportunity to ensure the child receives an adequate and varied diet in order to promote health and growth. However, the patterns of movement of the lips, tongue and jaw, when coordinating with breathing for eating and drinking will also influence the development of movements necessary for speech and saliva control (Chailey Heritage 1998). In addition the opportunity is there to develop posture, head control and hand–eye coordination; communication skills and learning the rules of social interaction, cultural and religious customs; and finally by offering choices and control the child will develop self-control and independence.

The development of eating and drinking patterns from infancy

Learning to eat is something that most of us take for granted, but it is a complex process. It depends on intact structures and function of the anatomy of the oral cavity and pharynx (Stevenson and Allaire 1996). Feeding begins as a reflex and becomes a voluntary act with only the pharyngeal and oesophageal stages remaining reflexive.

Every infant has to coordinate breathing, sucking and swallowing and tends to gag easily. This is because their anatomy is different to adults in that the tongue is relatively large and fills the mouth, and there is only room for a nipple/teat and a liquid diet. As the infant grows and develops and the neck lengthens, the space between the tongue and the sides and roof of the mouth widens, the gag reflex gradually recedes to the posterior third of the tongue (Alexander 1991) and since the tongue tip has more room to move, babbling may commence. Under normal circumstances it takes three years to learn eating and drinking skills and begins before birth.

In utero the foetus develops a curled position, adopting the elongated neck, head slightly forward and chin tucked in position that is important for eating. Thus the pre-term infant is already at a disadvantage not having been *in utero* sufficiently long to develop the curled position.

Deglutition or swallowing also occurs *in utero* from 16–17 weeks gestation (Walter 1994). By approximately six months of age the child has the head and trunk control necessary for good positioning as well as teeth with which to chew. However, chewing is neurologically determined, so that a mouth full of teeth does not necessarily mean chewing can take place. As the infant learns to roll over, so the transverse tongue reflex comes into action to roll food over the tongue. The phasic bite reflex now forms the basis of munching, the up and down movement, which the child has to learn to control to be able to bite and chew. It is not until the age of approximately 1 year that food is transferred from side to side without stopping in the middle of the tongue.

As the child learns to crawl, using diagonal movements, so the grinding, rotatory movement of the jaw develops to crush tougher foods, and as the child begins to walk and the hips rotate, the tongue also develops a rotatory movement and the child gradually learns to deal with different textures and combinations of food, having gained control of lip closure and cheek action (Milla 1991). Thus the development of eating skills is linked to gross motor development. As the child tries new textures the mouth gradually becomes desensitised and gagging is reduced. The longer a child is not experiencing things in the mouth, the longer it takes to learn not to gag. The sensory-motor play of infants is an important part of development that helps to desensitise the gag reflex, but some children may not be able to achieve this without help. Children with abnormal tone and hypersensitivity respond to the touch of food and utensils with increased muscle tone and abnormal oral patterns which make food intake very difficult and increase the risk of choking and vomiting (Sullivan and Rosenbloom 1996).

Contributory factors to learning eating/drinking skills

While growth and neurological maturation are very important for feeding development, experiential learning is also crucial. Children need to have the opportunity to try different food substances. Sensation and sensory feedback involving proprioception (feedback from muscles/joints and body awareness in space), touch, pressure, temperature and taste all contribute to learning to eat and swallow. New methods of food presentation may cause the child to revert to earlier patterns of movement e.g. when first given puréed food the infant will suck it from the spoon. Thus it is only with experience that children learn to deal qualitatively with different types of food substances in different ways (Stevenson and Allaire 1996).

Other important influences on learning to eat are fine motor development, methods of food presentation and cognitive development (Stevenson and Allaire 1996).

Critical period of learning

Pre-term infants and those with central nervous system dysfunction may require prolonged enteral or parenteral feeding and thus be deprived of oral stimulation for prolonged periods. These children may be resistant to oral feedings and have great difficulty learning to take nutrition by mouth. It has been suggested that there is a critical period for learning these skills and that after this period a particular behaviour can no longer be learned (Illingsworth and Lister 1964). Although this concept has been described and studied in animals, it has not been extensively studied in humans and remains unproven. However, in the writer's experience there does seem to be a point where the child will not rather than cannot learn eating and drinking skills. It is therefore a challenge to professionals to try and overcome these difficulties. There is no reason why weaning an infant with disabilities should not commence between 4–7 months of age, the same as for a child without disabilities. The only difference is that it may take much longer and will require a great amount of patience and perseverance.

Cup drinking also needs to be introduced early on (Carroll and Reilly 1996), in order for the infant to move on from the immature tongue movements used during suckling, and to develop the oral muscles and more mature rotatory tongue movements necessary for speech development as well as chewing and swallowing.

Meeting nutritional needs

As Chailey Heritage (1998) suggest, balancing nutritional needs with physical, developmental, behavioural, emotional and social needs is always difficult if not impossible without compromise. However, nutritional needs cannot be compromised without affecting the child's health and well-being. An inadequate diet may result in apathy, constipation, lack of concentration, poor wound healing, slow growth and physical development, decreased appetite and reduced resistance to infection. It is important, therefore, to discuss the nutritional needs of the individual infant/child with the dietician, so that an appropriate intake can be identified.

The mature swallowing process

Physiologically there are four stages to developing a mature swallowing process: oral preparatory stage; oral stage; pharyngeal stage; and oesophageal stage. However, Chailey Heritage (1998) reminds us that there is an anticipatory stage involving the sight, smell, taste, and texture of the meal or snack. This is particularly important to consider for the child with a sensory impairment.

The mature swallow may be studied in greater depth elsewhere (Walter 1994; Stevenson and Allaire 1996; Chailey Heritage 1998). Briefly however, the oral preparatory stage is concerned with getting food and fluid into the mouth. This requires the use of the lips and/or teeth for removing food from a fork or spoon. The oral stage prepares the food for swallowing and involves tongue and jaw activity to pass the semi-solid bolus of food to the back of the mouth. These two stages are voluntary, unlike the final two, which are involuntary. The pharyngeal stage involves the tongue and walls of the throat to transport the bolus to the oesophagus. If this is poorly timed it may result in coughing and choking which is a protective action to prevent food and drink entering the windpipe and lungs. Finally the oesophageal stage consists of the automatic transfer of the bolus to the stomach. For the child with disabilities, depending on their specific difficulties, there may be problems during any or all of these stages.

Exercise

For the reader to see for him/herself how these stages operate the following exercise may help.
Drink a small amount of water from a cup and then a spoon, and eat a biscuit. Do this at normal speed and then again in slow motion and notice how you deal with the food and fluid and which part of the mouth is most involved at each stage (Mencap 1994). Also notice how you think about and anticipate eating, use your eyes and nose, and notice how you breathe and how you sit (Chailey Heritage 1998).

Why feeding difficulties occur

The early feeding of some children with disabilities may be difficult due to abnormal or absent reflexes. Conversely persistent reflexes may limit voluntary movements and control. Thus children who have experienced early difficulties such as prolonged tube feeding, and have not been able to enjoy and be comforted by eating experiences, may be distressed by the first experience of food and drink being given by mouth (Goldbart *et al.* 1994).

Abnormal structure of the mouth, tongue and jaw e.g. cleft lip and palate, and sometimes the delayed or abnormal appearance of teeth, may also interfere with feeding. Some other difficulties are listed in Table 8.1.

Table 8.1 Problems that may interfere with eating

1. Disorders of muscle tone affecting general posture and the posture and movements of the jaw, lips and tongue.
2. Oral reflexes may be absent, develop late, be exaggerated or persist for a much longer period.
3. The child may be hypersensitive to touch or may be unaware of the presence of food in the mouth – hypo- or hypersensitive gag response.
4. Problems with the heart, digestive system or respiratory system may lead to failure to thrive and a period of nasogastric tube feeding.
5. Metabolic disorders or food allergies.
6. Insufficient motor skills to cope with different textures or consistency of food.
7. Physical or inflammatory conditions affecting the oesophagus causing food to be associated with pain and discomfort e.g. gastro-oesophageal reflux.
8. Behavioural problems e.g. frequent vomiting during/after meals or spitting out lumps originating from previous physical problems which have been resolved.
9. The continued use of a particular utensil may lead to a persistent pattern of behaviour e.g. a spouted trainer cup maintaining a suckle-drinking pattern.
10. Inconsistent handling leading to problems in establishing new feeding patterns and routines e.g. different management at home and at school.
11. Visual impairment and deafness.
12. Constipation.
13. Impaired hand function.
14. Dental problems.
15. Communication difficulties.

General points to consider

It is important to remember that each child has individual needs that need assessing by the multi-disciplinary team. However, there are some universal approaches, such as ensuring the child's position is stable and secure and is maintained throughout the meal. This will contribute to the development of head control and hand/eye coordination, which are necessary for competent eating and drinking (Chailey Heritage 1998). For the child in the acute setting it may be necessary to ask the parents to bring in their special seating or standing system to ensure the child's positioning is correct, not only for mealtimes, but also for play. Sitting in a wheelchair all the time, for instance, may not be appropriate.

Another point to remember is that oral reactions, which affect feeding patterns, may be stimulated by temperature, taste, thickness and texture of the food and fluid (Chailey Heritage 1998). Thus extremes of temperature, strong flavours and smells may stimulate a reaction. Thicker fluids are generally easier to control since they slow the flow, enabling more control.

In the acute hospital setting the personal profile/communication passport mentioned (see Chapter 9) can provide essential information on helping the disabled child meet their nutritional needs. It is an extremely useful tool to ensure that both professional and non-professional carers can meet the daily care needs of the child with disabilities. However, for children who do not have a personal communication passport/profile it will be important to remember to ask the family some vital questions:

- What are the child's likes and dislikes related to food?
- What is the preferred temperature of the food?
- What is the preferred texture of food?
- Preferred pace – is the child a fast or slow eater?
- Does the child need to be in a distraction-free environment, i.e. free from noise from TVs and other background noises?
- Is there anything else that may be relevant?

Equipment

The child's physiotherapist and occupational therapist (OT) are the professionals to liaise with regarding the appropriate seating or standing frame to ensure their optimal position for meal and snack times. The pelvis and trunk need to be stable, the child's feet flat on the floor and their forearms resting on the table (Chailey Heritage 1998). However, as previously stated, equipment brought in from home is likely to be the most suitable for use in the acute setting as it has already been correctly fitted to the child. Although space may well be a problem in a busy children's ward, the importance of this equipment in order to maintain the skills the child has already learnt cannot be over-emphasised. These skills may have taken many months, or even years of painstaking work by the child, family and professionals, to acquire, but may be lost very quickly if the child is not given the opportunity to utilise them whilst in hospital. Thus access to the right equipment can be seen to have a very significant effect, not only on how children eat and feed themselves, but also on their ability to maintain the skills they have acquired (Chailey Heritage 1998).

The child's OT and Speech and Language therapist (SALT) are the professionals who can advise on specialised cutlery to enable independent or assisted feeding e.g. an angled spoon and perhaps a high-sided plate to make it easier for the carer to load food onto the spoon (Chailey Heritage 1998).

There is a huge range of specialist equipment, which may help the child to be more independent. In an ideal world every children's ward would have a paediatric OT and a few selected items of equipment from which to choose for those children for whom it has not been possible to bring their own.

Prompts

Chailey Heritage (1998) suggests various prompts to prepare the child for eating and drinking. These include being able to see other people eating, providing a role model, and maybe also eliciting a feeling of being included. Being able to see and anticipate the arrival of the meal is also important so that for the visually impaired child, verbal prompts will be necessary. In any case it may be helpful to talk the child through the process and remind them of what they have to do, using phrases such as 'look', 'load the spoon', 'open mouth,' etc. Finally, physically prompting the child by offering a small amount of food enables them to be prepared for the taste, temperature and texture; while gently stroking the lower lip with the spoon may stimulate eating/drinking movement patterns.

Relationship between feeder and child being fed

A relaxed child, who knows and trusts their carer, will ensure that mealtimes are a more pleasurable experience. Knowing the child well means that the person feeding them will be more in tune with the child's communication, preferences and choices as well as method of feeding, utensils used and the preferred pace. Continuity in service providers should lead to satisfaction with care, adherence to recommendations and reduced stress and worry for the parents (King, King and Rosenbaum 1996). In the acute setting it may well be the student who is given the task of feeding the child with disabilities, due to the amount of time and preparation necessary. There may be little opportunity on a busy ward to build rapport, however, it is important to take some time to do so prior to the next mealtime, so that the child does not become overly anxious, and unable to enjoy their meal.

Some points to consider when preparing to assist a child to eat and drink are included below in Table 8:2.

Table 8.2 Points to consider when preparing to assist a child to eat

- Is the child prepared for food? Is there pleasurable anticipation?
- Does the child share in the whole experience of feeding?
- Can they see the food arrive? See how it is presented? Can they smell the food?
- Is each mouthful prepared for verbally? Or with a 'taster' to trigger a response?
- Is the child given the opportunity to communicate and indicate choice? By eye pointing, using symbols/photographs, signs or other communication aids?

Behavioural problems

Many children demonstrate difficult behaviour at mealtimes such as refusing food, being fussy over what they eat, spitting out food, vomiting, playing with food or poor appetite. Providing food for children is a very emotionally charged activity (Chailey Heritage 1998), and any behaviour problems may arouse feelings of failure, frustration, anger and resentment in the carer. Although the carer may find it hurtful, refusal to eat is not necessarily a personal rejection.

Croft (1992) showed that children with severe oral-motor dysfunction, can take 6–18 times longer to eat a mouthful of food than normal children. Therefore feeding the disabled child can be unrewarding. However, provided the child's overall nutrition is adequate, one meal or even poor intake over a whole day may not have a significant impact on their overall state of nutrition. The situation does, however, require careful monitoring in order to ensure the child's nutritional status is maintained.

Care-givers' needs

Ensuring one's own needs are addressed before beginning the task of feeding a child is vital, if interruptions are to be avoided. Taking a few moments to consider the questions listed in Table 8.3 may be helpful in ensuring both your own needs and those of the child are met.

Roles of the 'feeding' team

From the above it can be deduced that the differing aspects of providing the optimum conditions to enable a child to enjoy mealtimes, while meeting their nutritional requirements and improving their self-help skills, all overlap. Table 8.4 shows the roles of the multi-disciplinary team members who may be involved.

Conclusion

Considerable thought and preparation is necessary before beginning to feed the child with disabilities. This chapter has attempted to provide the reader with some ideas of what questions they need to be asking, both of

Table 8.3 Preparing yourself and the child for the task of eating and drinking

- Do you need to go to the loo?
- Are you pushed for time – if so could someone else be asked to assist with feeding or take over the urgent task?
- Do you have everything you need?
- Have you somewhere comfortable to sit?
- Is it right for the person you are assisting to feed?
- Can you be focused on the person you are assisting?
- Is the environment distraction free? The child may have difficulty sifting out important things from the irrelevant.
- Can you minimise noise from TV or radio? Or preferably turn them off.
- What are others doing in the same area?
- Is the light right?
- Is the room temperature too hot/cold?
- Does the child have suitable communication aids available?
- Can the service be flexible enough to meet the needs of the child?
- If meals are best little and often can this need be met?
- Are extra resources available?
- How is information relating to assistance with feeding passed on?
- Does the child have a personal profile?
- Is the child comfortable and in the right position for eating/drinking?
- Do they need toileting or changing?
- How do they feel? – Are they happy, tired, sad, in discomfort or pain?
- What choices and control do they have?
- What, When, Where will they eat?
- Is their head in the midline to enable them to concentrate?
- Who will assist them?
- Which other service users are present or next to them?

Table 8.4 The roles of the multi-disciplinary team

speech and language therapist	oral competence
paediatrician	physical health and well-being
physiotherapist	positioning and handling
occupational therapist	position, equipment and self-feeding
dietician	nutrition
dentist	dentition
child and adolescent psychologist	emotional and behavioural problems
children's nurse	implementer of action plans, co-ordinators, teacher and support to parents

themselves, and of the 'feeding' team should they have any concerns about what they are doing. Assisting a child to eat and drink requires the carer to be totally focused on what they are doing and therefore also requires their ability to recognise and meet their own needs prior to commencing the task. Continuity of care to ensure a relaxed and happy child, as well as a good relationship with the family is not a luxury but essential, in order to provide high quality care. This will, no doubt, have implications for staffing levels so that neither the child nor the person assisting them will feel pressured to complete the task as fast as possible. The child with disabilities needs to feel secure and comfortable with the person assisting them in order to be able to respond to them. The writer has observed from experience that it can take many months to get to know a child well and for the child to begin to respond and that the amount of time available in the acute setting is not always conducive to building relationships. However, since many children with disabilities may well have frequent admissions to hospital, it may be possible for the same staff to care for them on subsequent admissions and provide some continuity. The increasing use of personal profiles for these children will help to give families confidence that their child's needs will be met even in their absence.

References

Alexander, R. (1991) 'Pre-Speech and Feeding', in J. L. Bigge (ed.) *Teaching Individuals with Multiple Disabilities*, New York: Macmillan.

Carpenter, B. (1997) *Families in Context: Emerging Trends in Family Support and Early Intervention*, London: Fulton.

Carroll, L. and Reilly, S. (1996)'The therapeutic approach to the child with feeding difficulties', in P. Sullivan and L. Rosenbloom (eds) *Feeding the Disabled Child*, London: MacKeith Press.

Chailey Heritage (1998) *Eating and Drinking Skills for Children with Motor Disorders*, Chailey Heritage Clinical Services.

Croft, R. D. (1992) 'What consistency of food is best for children with cerebral palsy who cannot chew', *Archives of Disease in Childhood*, 67, 269–271.

Goldbart, J., Warner, J. and Mount, H. (1994) *The Development of Early Communication and Feeding – A workshop training package*, Manchester: Mencap.

Illingsworth, R. S. and Lister, J. (1964) 'The Critical or Sensitive Period, with special reference to certain problems in infants and children', *Journal of Paediatrics*, 65, 839–848.

King, G., King, S. M., Rosenbaum, P. L. (1996) 'Interpersonal aspects of care-giving and client outcomes: A review of the Literature', *Ambulatory Child Health*, 2, 151–160.

Laverty, H. and Reet, M. (2000a) *Hello this is Me, Care Planning Documentation*, London: Jessica Kingsley.

Laverty, H. and Reet, M. (2000b) *Hello this is Me, Assessment and Independency Rating Tool*, London: Jessica Kingsley.

Milla, P. J. (1991) 'Feeding, Tasting and Sucking', in W. A. Walker, P. R. Durie, J. A. Hamilton, J. A. Walker Smith and J. B. Watkins (eds) *Pediatric Gastrointestinal Disease*, Philadelphia: B.C. Declan.

Stevenson, R. and Allaire, J. (1996) 'The Development of Eating Skills in Infants and Young Children', in P. Sullivan and L. Rosenbloom, *Feeding the Disabled Child*, London: MacKeith.

Sullivan, P. B. and Rosenbloom, L. (1996) *Feeding the Disabled Child*, London: MacKeith.

Tippett, A. (2001) 'All About Me: Documentation for Children with Special Needs', *Paediatric Nursing*, 13(10) December, 34–35.

Walter, R. M. D. (1994) 'Issues Surrounding the Development of Feeding and Swallowing', chapter 2 in D. Tuchman and R. Walter (eds) *Disorders of Feeding and Swallowing in Infants and Children*, California: Singular.

Warner, H. (2000) 'Making the Invisible, Visible', *Journal Child Health Care* 4(3) Autumn, 123–126.

9 Finding a mechanism for communication

Helen K. Warner

This chapter will discuss how and why we communicate and what we can do to enable the severely disabled child to make their needs known if they are unable to use language. There will be a section on how we enhance the learning of language within the Early Intervention Unit and what other means of communication may be used where language is slow to develop or may not be an option. Finally suggestions will be made as to what can be done in the acute setting, such as the use of personal profiles, to ensure that the child's basic human needs for control, respect and support (King, King and Rosenbaum 1996) are met.

Learning to communicate

Learning to communicate verbally is the most complex skill that human beings develop. Under normal circumstances language is learned within 5 years, progressing from the use of non-verbal messages to using verbal communication and the spoken word. Learning about communication begins at birth, the first year being critical for the foundations to be laid and for non-verbal communication to develop i.e. the use of eye contact and development of turn-taking to signal a joint focus of attention. Even when the talking begins, there is still a great deal to learn, and it takes years to refine and perfect the use of language until eventually it becomes grammatically and phonologically correct.

> It takes two to talk . . . what we do as adults and how we do it, will affect a child's opportunities to learn how to communicate.
>
> (Manolson 1992: 3)

Two-way communication can only develop where there are frequent interactions between children and, initially, their carers and later their peers. Thus the importance of opportunities to mix with their peers at an early age cannot be over-emphasised. During the interactions with their carers children need to be provided with relevant information appropriate to their level of understanding, so that it can be used to build on what they already know.

How and why language develops

Weitzman (1992) describes seven stages of normal language development from birth to age 5 years, although children with developmental delays may take longer to achieve each stage. The first stage is reflexive, the infant having no understanding that his behaviour can affect others and cause them to behave in certain ways. Infants respond to their bodily needs and to the environment, for example, they cry when hungry or startled by a noise. By responding to the infant's actions and sounds the carer enables the infant to feel loved and secure and to begin to anticipate that his/her needs will be met.

From 6–8 weeks of age the infant gradually begins to make cooing noises when relaxed and settled. Talking to him/her will get him to coo in response and when face to face with his main carer. As the baby and adult smile at each other and make cooing noises to each other, the foundations for two-way interactions are laid. Before the age of 6 months, interaction is in the form of mutual gaze. Coupe and Goldbart (1988) describe levels of eye contact which need to develop, and emphasise the fact that communication in the form of gaze happens for different functions, e.g. requests, and comments, in the absence of words.

Baby and care-giver spend time together where the adult talks and leaves gaps for the baby to fill using vocalisations. The baby's actions are taken as a response in dialogue. Communication at this stage remains largely pre-intentional and relies on the adult interpreting the behaviour as if there is a reason for behaving in a specific way. Carer studies (Snow 1977) indicate that prior to age 6 months, parents will accept everything the infant does/says as meaningful communication, the mother leading and directing the inter-actions, which gradually increase in 'demand and content'. After age 6 months, the carer begins to shape the child's responses so that they will respond only to specific vocalisations. Thus by only accepting more clearly defined behaviours as communicative, parents build and shape intentional communication. As the child begins to reach out for objects it becomes easier to interpret what it is that is wanted and also to interpret the sounds, facial expressions and body movements that indicate pleasure, displeasure, anger, contentment and enthusiasm.

Babbling happens early on at the pre-intentional communication level, as the baby begins to experiment with sound and he/she will make noises to themselves in a mirror as well as having 'conversations' with their carer. Vowel sounds come first and as the child gains more control over his/her body, consonants/vowel combinations will be heard. The child will experiment with all sounds including those not used in their own language sound system e.g. African clicks and pharyngeals. The child enjoys games such as peek-a-boo and will smile happily, letting the adult know they want more by making sounds or moving their body and thus taking their turn.

Interest in toys/objects increases and eye contact may temporarily decrease until the child is able to coordinate looking both at their carer and the toy they are playing with. At this stage they do not understand words but only the non-verbal cues such as gestures, intonation and the general situation. Language takes time to learn, but even when a child cannot yet talk, he is learning to connect and communicate (Manolson 1992). Words need to be heard, understood, copied and repeated many times before they become part of the child's vocabulary. The words will initially be situation-specific although the child will also experiment with words outside the situation in which they are learned. Children will gradually progress from using gestures to using sounds, which become clearer and more precise with practice. From the use of single words, children progress to phrases, sentences and finally to the use of correct grammar at a much later stage. If the adult caring for them talks about what is happening or going to happen, in familiar situations, the child will learn from his experiences, but it will be contextual understanding, the child not yet understanding the words beyond the context. Also, if the adult interprets what the child may be feeling, in those situations, the child will have the opportunity to hear the appropriate words so that he can use them when he needs to.

Use of facial expressions and gestures will help children to understand the words used and show them a way of expressing themselves before being able to talk. This is also why children are responsive to action songs, which provide physical clues to the meaning being communicated. Constant repetition of key words and sounds every time children are played with, will make it easier for them to focus on new words and sounds by association with what is happening to them, leading to anticipation of what comes next.

Children with disabilities

Since experience comes first, followed by understanding and finally language, children with physical and learning disabilities are clearly at a disadvantage when it comes to learning language (Manolson 1992). The child with physical disabilities may have limited experiences and therefore opportunities to learn, because of delays in their gross motor skills and being unable to reach out for toys/objects of interest. They may also have problems with their auditory and visual processing skills, such as attention and memory, and poor integration of their multi-sensory input (Kot and Law 1995).

The child's position will also affect the type of movement that they are able to make in order to communicate e.g. holding their head in the midline enabling looking, reaching and vocalising. Similarly the child with learning disability may find difficulty in understanding that their facial, vocal, gestures, and other behaviours have an effect on others to bring about social interaction and gratification of needs. Thus they may remain in Piaget's (1975) sensory-motor stage of development, which is the stage of pre-intentional communication. This means that they do not actively intend to communicate, but their carers can interpret their emotional responses such as enjoyment, dislike, and states of alertness to various events, placing meanings on the child's expressions (Coupe *et al.* 1985). These children may demonstrate fewer and poorer affective behaviours for care-givers to build on. This means that two-way communication will not occur spontaneously and opportunities with appropriate support may need to be provided in order to move towards this goal. Thus the child's carers need to be 'tuned in' and sensitive to any signals/messages the child is making, and to respond to them appropriately in ways that will increase the frequency and occurrence of these behaviours so that the child is enabled to develop and strengthen potentially communicative 'signals' (Coupe *et al.* 1985).

The emphasis, when interacting with the child, should be on waiting and allowing the child sufficient time to respond. Often care-givers of children with special needs will have altered boundaries and tend to be very protective, so that spontaneous interaction does not always happen (Wood *et al.* 1976; Jones 1981; Bondurant *et al.* 1983). The child's needs may be anticipated by their carers, who may not be allowing the child to influence his/her environment as much as they could by underestimating the amount of time necessary to allow this to happen. Some profoundly handicapped children with cerebral palsy, for instance, were found not to know how to choose because they had never been given the opportunity to choose (Evans-Morris 1981). Thus the ability of the child to interact is reliant on the adults caring for them being aware of the child's non-verbal behaviours and responding to them in a consistent way.

In the Early Intervention Unit

The first step towards enhancing the communication skills of the developmentally delayed child is to observe and assess the child's behaviours in given situations, during play, so that potentially communicative behaviours may be identified. Often, behaviours will be displayed which are due to frustration because there is no other way the child can communicate. With time and patience it is possible to discover what the child will respond to and what he/she will turn away from, and, their unique combination of body language and sounds used to communicate (Manolson 1992). Music can be a highly effective facilitator for improving physical movement, and feeding, as well as communication and language skills. It can contribute to a reduction in hyperactivity, increased body awareness and improvement in cognitive and communication development (Morris and Klein 1998).

Once a motivator has been identified, the staff can then respond consistently during the daily routine, and the environment can be adapted to present opportunities for the child to affect it and to initiate communication, however inadvertently. As with any child at this stage of development it is important to imitate their own sounds or facial expressions and particularly important to give them time to respond. The amount of time will be individual to the child, but will be much longer than for the typical child as it will take them longer to process the information before considering an appropriate response. If inadequate time is allowed for the infant/child to respond they may well lose interest and not bother to try, and the opportunity for the child to learn is lost.

The Early Intervention Unit provides an enriched environment, which is supported by a speech and language therapist to maximise the opportunities for children to learn, while simultaneously being part of the assessment process. In the unit an air of expectancy is the norm. Expectancy is goal free and has been described by Weitzman (1992) as a feeling of excitement and anticipation that something wonderful will happen or be discovered. Thus although the final goal is unclear the process itself is the focus of care, allowing children to make discoveries and learn along the way. Having a facilitative environment allows children to discover choices and new ways of being and encourages the families to believe that their child can learn and achieve his/her true potential, whatever that may be.

The staff can begin to challenge the tragedy of belief systems that impose limitations on what the individual child may achieve and thus also begin to break down the negative fears that can create a barrier to the child's learning.

Frequent intensive interactions (Nind and Hewett 1995) are made as the children are able to tolerate them. Smith (1989: 113) summarised what care-givers/parents do in this extremely responsive process:

> They arrange, manipulate and structure the environment in order to facilitate and maximise children's interactions. They do this by making use of the children's interests and inclinations, and most importantly by being very sensitive to feedback from the children in determining what to select as the focus of joint attention.

This means that the adult is attentive and focused within a relaxed and informal setting, demonstrating acceptance of whatever the child is doing, so that the child will feel confident to continue to produce more behaviours. Imitating or 'modified reflecting' is a good way to celebrate the child's behaviour (Nind and Hewett 1995). In these interactions the adult and child are equal, the adult being available as a 'reassuring interpreter' of the child's world. In this way the child will learn that being with other people is good and that he himself is good to be with.

Mealtimes can provide a high level of need and motivation to communicate, and are used to incorporate important concepts such as turn taking and the roles of initiator and responder. For example, waiting for a signal to put the spoon into the child's mouth, and signals for a pause or different food all indicate the child is initiating an interaction. If there can be a variety of small dishes of food, the child has more opportunity to make choices rather than if the whole meal is all on one plate. The only limits are the food available and the carer's imagination.

Children within the unit are encouraged to use objects of reference such as being shown a cup at drink time or a ball for ball-play. As they begin to make the association the children begin to anticipate what is coming next so that any frustration is reduced. Makaton, a sign and symbol system, helps the message to reach the brain by using another sense so that the meaning of a word is illustrated and the children learn through the action. This approach is used to reinforce the spoken word and is often imitated by the children before the words begin to be used. Children with autism, and some other diagnoses, are taught to use objects of reference and also the picture exchange communication system (PECS). This is a system of communication whereby the child learns to give a picture of what he wants to an adult who then rewards him/her with the object he/she is asking for.

A child's gross motor and fine motor skills will affect their ability to communicate, the development of all these skills being interlinked and inseparable. Within the early intervention nursery the opportunity to learn through play is critical to enhance development in all areas.

The important opportunity for children to mix and interact with their peers is also provided. Interacting with peers impacts on both social and language development, and enables children to see things from another's perspective, to compromise, resolve conflicts, share, collaborate and cooperate with others (Weitzman 1992). Another important skill, for the children, is learning to negotiate and to assert themselves. If children do not have the language or social skills to interact with their peers they will be left out and unable to learn the skills normally learned. Providing opportunities to allow interactions to take place with peers will therefore help to lay the foundations for further learning to take place, while satisfying the child's emotional need to belong.

Personal profiles

In the Nursery, families are encouraged to write a personal profile/communication passport to enable the professionals to gain a clearer picture of who the child is. The purpose of a personal profile is to gather a range of information about an individual who has difficulty communicating their needs and desires to others, so that the information can be considered when working with or interacting with the individual. There is often an 'information gap' where many people hold a great deal of important and useful information about the individual but it is not accessible to everyone involved. Thus the profile is a way of bridging that gap and helping everyone get to know the individual more fully so that their needs may be met more effectively.

Personal profiles/communication passports have been found to be most effective and meaningful when written in the first person (Stanislawski 1997; Tippett 2001; Catalano *et al.* 2002; Millar and Aitken 2003). The information is presented in a clear, concise and positive manner.

Close observation allows parents to identify their child's own likes/dislikes. Putting ourselves into the child's shoes enables us to gain insight into how he is feeling and how we can best provide intervention, and by observing the child we can learn more about his/her strengths and weaknesses (Catalano *et al.* 2002). All the information necessary to meet the child's needs on a daily basis is included in the profile.

Initially a sample profile is given to parents, with some questions to prompt their responses. The family are helped to complete the profile to ensure that nothing relevant is left out. This can be therapeutic for families as it helps them to focus on the positive aspects of their child, while allowing those who read the profile to gain some insight into how well they are accepting and adapting to their child's circumstances. Families are encouraged to include photographs and drawings and to make the profile as personal as they like. The profile is then put into a clear, loose-leaf binder and remains the property of the family. It is, however, impressed upon the family that this is only the beginning and simply a snapshot of their child. In order for it to be useful, it will need to be regularly reviewed and updated, as the child grows and develops and learns new skills, so that it always reflects how the child is in the present. At the end of each profile is a section to allow anyone who reads it to sign and put his/her comments or requests for further information as necessary. In this way they can help to ensure that new information is continually added and updated. Additional information that may need to be added may include information relating to feelings, relationships, triggers and behavioural strategies, achievements and aims/dreams for the future.

The nursery staff will also come to know the children well and can add their own observations on how the child behaves in the nursery environment. In this way a more complete and balanced view of the child is put together over a period of time. Wherever the child goes, the profile should go too, as it is the voice of the child to help make their needs and wishes known and understood. Thus they may be of use to wider family members, pre-school units and schools and also the acute setting, and may give confidence to parents that their child's needs can be consistently met even in their absence. Table 9.1 is an example of the profile contents.

Ways of using a personal profile

Using a profile can help us better understand the child and therefore to be more empathetic of his/her behaviours. Sharing the profile with teachers, therapists, family members and doctors will ensure the child's behaviours, needs, feelings, likes and dislikes are communicated, to improve his quality of life, while enabling the professionals to identify reasons for a specific behaviour and to work out an effective strategy to deal with it. When parents, care-givers and professionals work together as a team to generate answers to the questions raised by the profile a transdisciplinary understanding of the child is promoted (Warner 2001). Profiles may also be used for teaching purposes in a variety of situations e.g. by professionals for other professionals, and also in schools, to allow a child's classmates to understand

Table 9.1 Example of Profile content

Hello—My Name is:
About Me—birth history, SCBU
My Family—who I live with, plus emergency telephone numbers
Other important people/pets in my life (plus professionals involved)
More about Me—personality, usual routine, naptimes, regular medications,
can I see and hear well? Do I wear glasses? hearing aid? etc. What comforts me if
I'm unhappy?
Eating and Drinking—mealtime routines, equipment, food temperature preferred,
fast or slow eater, likes/dislikes
Communication—How I communicate/ Feelings/ Behavioural strategies
Likes/Dislikes—toys, music, hugs, how I like to be held, carried, move around
Toileting—nappies, potty training
What I can do—eye contact, tracking, head control, roll, sit independently etc.
If I am not happy this checklist may help (too hot? too cold? Need a cuddle/ drink
etc.)
Have I forgotten anything?
Autographs and comments
A sample of the above is given to parents together with a letter addressed to the child,
asking them to enlist the help of their parents to put the relevant information
together so that nursery staff can help the child to settle in more quickly.

---

their peer's behaviour and be encouraged to interact with him/her. The profile is also a record of the child's life and contains facts about the child that may otherwise be forgotten. They are therefore a useful reminder to look back on and see how far the child has come when changes are difficult to perceive and may be subtle.

Augmentative and alternative communication

Even when children have complex communication difficulties, communication is possible and essential (Morris 1999). For children and young people who may be unable to communicate in conventional ways, other suitable means of communication must be found, and since in most circumstances, adults control the means of communication for children with disabilities, it is important that they are aware of the alternative methods available.

Augmentative and alternative communication (AAC) refers to any method of communication that supplements the usual methods of speech and handwriting when these are not an option. The United Nations Convention on the Rights of the Child (1989) recognises that children have a right to obtain information and to express their opinions and have those opinions taken into account in any procedure that may affect them. The use of AACs can enhance the quality of children's lives, allowing them to access education, increase independence and allow them to participate more fully in society.

Since children are individual in their needs an accurate assessment of which method or combination of methods will work for them is essential and should be carried out by a speech and language therapist. There are various systems available to meet a wide range of needs and skill levels (Rumble and Larcher 1998). Most AAC users employ a number of different forms of AAC depending on the situation, and may include a combination of unaided and aided communication systems which may be low or highly technical aids (see Tables 9.2 and 9.3). Consideration of the individual child's cognitive and language levels will need to be taken into account when deciding on an appropriate communication aid.

According to Millar and Scott (1998), identifying the most appropriate AAC system and finding funding appears to be relatively easy. The funding comes from the government and a local assessment is carried out, by suitably qualified people, including a speech therapist, to ensure the child's needs are appropriately met. The difficulty is in ensuring effective use of the system and integrating it into daily life, at home, school and at work.

In the acute setting

> One of the most disrespectful things that can be done to an individual is to fail to communicate with, and thus relate to, that person in a style which that person can comprehend.
>
> (Nind and Hewett 1995: 174)

This statement underpins how important it is that, when a child is admitted to the acute setting, the nurse discovers the level at which the child understands events and experiences around them. The parents are the primary

Table 9.2 Low-tech communication aids

Pointer boards/photographs
Switches
Signing and symbol systems e.g. Makaton
Cued speech, lip reading, objects of reference
Blissymbolics, Rebus, PECS
Tactile systems e.g. Braille, Moon, Deaf-Blind Manual Alphabet

Table 9.3 High-tech communication aids

- Computer based communication equipment.
- High-tech aids can be adapted to be operated by minimal movements such as a single switch press that can be used by the severely physically disabled individual.
- Communication systems with synthesised or digitalised voice – for those who cannot speak. (However, these require a good knowledge of language, social skills and understanding in order to work).
- Enlarged displays or voice feedback offer computer access to those with visual impairments. (The child needs to have an understanding of words).

source of this information but where this is not available the child's school may provide the information required.

Useful information can be gained by completing the statements below during the nursing assessment. Obtaining this information will allow the nursing staff to communicate with the child at a time when they may be feeling distress and discomfort and enable their involvement in the caring process, rather than assuming what their needs are and how those needs may be met.

Communicating with me
I usually/sometimes/rarely understand events and experience . . .
I usually communicate by using . . .
I can tell you by . . .
If I am in discomfort or pain I can tell you by . . .
If I like something I . . .
If I don't like something I . . .
If I like something, and want more I . . .
If I don't like something and want you to stop I . . .
I can use the following symbols or means of communication . . .

Adapted from Hutchfield and Parsons (2003)

However, it is worth, first asking if the child has a personal profile which will contain this information and can reduce the number of questions necessary to ask parents, who may be worried and anxious when their child is sick. Hospital admissions are potentially damaging to children (Bowlby 1971; Robertson 1970) and in particular to children with special needs (Warner 2000). The acute setting is not always conducive to enhancing the children's development and communication behaviours in the same way that they are enhanced in the early intervention nursery, and it is not so easy to adapt the environment for the child. Chronic shortages of experienced staff also mean that often these children are looked after by junior staff, who may not have sufficient knowledge or experience of caring for children with disabilities. They may also have difficulty finding enough time to fully meet the child's needs due to having to prioritise the acutely ill children. However, in the same way that nurses need to be totally focused on the child when assisting them to eat and drink, it is also necessary to be focused when communicating with them, or the subtle behaviours displayed by the child may be easily missed.

In the acute setting nurses are at a disadvantage, often having little time to get to know the child's own subtle communication behaviours before they have to communicate with them as part of their nursing care. This may be all the more difficult if the child is feeling unwell or in pain, and may be frightened in an unfamiliar situation, all of which will affect his ability to communicate.

Nurses' own communication skills therefore become crucial to put families at ease, and to gain their confidence and trust while discovering the information they require regarding the child's communication abilities. Of equal importance is the need for nurses to be honest and admit to parents if they have not previously looked after a child with such complex needs. Positively learning from parents' expert knowledge of their child, while respecting their need for information about what to expect during their child's admission will go some way towards giving them back some control over their lives which, to reiterate is a basic human need (King, King, and Rosenbaum 1996).

Nurses can help to ensure the child is respected as an individual by demonstrating acceptance. Allowing all the health professionals involved the opportunity to look first at the child's profile before attempting to interact with him/her, will enable them to begin to understand the child's complex requirements and avoid making assumptions about the child's abilities.

Thus if the child uses an AAC it must be both available and also used. Opportunities to interact such as at mealtimes, playtimes, and any other time when nursing interventions or care needs have to be implemented, must be used therapeutically so that the child can practise what he has already learnt. In this way the child's ability to communicate can be maintained and the risk of losing skills already learned, minimised. If children are not given opportunities to communicate and affect their environment then they may well lose interest in trying to do so, thus undoing the work that has gone into them gaining the skills they already have and which may have taken them many months, or even years, to acquire.

The following play activities will encourage the child to gain control of his lips, tongue and soft palate, all of which play a part in speech sound production. The lips are also important for the control of dribbling, swallowing and blowing, and the tongue is also important for chewing, licking and swallowing. Although it is difficult to see the soft palate, which is a continuation of the hard palate (or roof of the mouth), and how well it moves, its function is to move up against the back of the throat and close off the nasal passages to prevent air moving up from the lungs and up into the nasal cavity. If it does not function well any speech produced will have a nasal tone. The soft palate also assumes this position during sucking and blowing activities. Opportunities that encourage a child to use the lips, tongue and soft palate can be fun while also enabling them to learn how to control them.

Suggested materials

Candles, bubbles, straws, whistles, blow pipes, cotton wool, tissue paper, ping pong balls, lipstick, paint and mirrors.

Suggested activities

(Adapted from the Advice Sheets for Parents: the Nuffield Hearing and Speech Centre)

- Use a mirror and encourage him/her to copy an 'oo' shape. At first, you may need to gently push the lips from a tight stretch position to the round position.

- Push lips forwards as for kissing. Practise kissing a teddy/dolly.
- Paint lips with lipstick and make round prints on paper or a mirror. Lip printing can also be done with lips together and also with a wide smile.
- Carnival blowers/whistles with rounded mouth-pieces to encourage lip rounding to be held with the lips and not the teeth.
- Hold a pencil between upper lips and nose – good for older children.
- Candles – use small cake candles stuck in something steady e.g. plasticine. Light the candles and encourage the child to gently blow them out. Alternatively try blowing out the candles through a straw. Blow the candles out slowly one at a time or aim for long blows by attempting to blow them all out together.
- Bubbles can be blown through the plastic wand or through a straw to produce many small bubbles. Also try blowing bubbles in a drink with a straw.
- Try blow-football using straws and ping pong balls. Cotton wool and tissue paper can be used in the same way.
- Blow paper fish into a pond. Also try using a straw.
- Blow painting – place a small blob of paint in the centre of a large piece of paper and blow the paint through a straw to produce a pattern.
- Try holding air under pressure in mouth e.g. blow out cheeks and explode air through the lips, or hold nose with fingers and blow. While blowing try to remove fingers and maintain the air stream through the mouth.
- Practise changing from a round shape to a spread lip shape e.g. pretend to be a goldfish for a round shape and then smile like a clown to produce a spread shape.
- Alternate kissing (with rounded lips) and smiling at (with lips spread) a teddy/dolly.
- Look in a mirror and encourage him/her to copy you sticking out your tongue or trying to touch your nose.
- Try everyday activities such as licking lollies, ice-cream, gummed paper, stars, envelopes etc.

For those children who are learning to speak but may have limited understanding it may be necessary to simplify our speech as we would with a very young child in the following ways:

- Emphasise the content words.
- Exaggerate pitch and intensity (Imagine talking to a baby in a pram).
- Longer pauses between utterances.
- Simplified vocabulary – and emphasis on concrete words (not abstract), which are repeated . . . and repeated . . .

- Talk about the 'here and now'.
- Talk about what interests them.
- Ask questions but do not expect answers.
- If necessary rearrange word order to have important information first.

(Adapted from Franklin 1996)

References

Bondurant, J. L., Romeo, D. J. and Kretschmer, R. (1983) 'Language behaviours of mothers of children with normal and delayed language', *Language, Speech and Hearing Services in Schools*, 14, 233–242.

Bowlby, J. (1971) *Attachment and Loss*, Harmondsworth: Penguin.

Catalano, C., Hernandez, P. and Wolters, P. (2002) 'A child's self-statement – Who am I?', *Exceptional Parent*, April, 60–65.

Coupe, J., Barton, L., Barber, M., Collins, L., Levy, D. and Murphy, D. (1985) *Affective Communication Assessment*, Manchester: Melland School.

Coupe, J. and Goldbart, J. (1988) *Communication before Speech*, London: Chapman and Hall.

Evans-Morris, S. (1981) 'Communication/interaction development at mealtimes for the multiply handicapped child: Implications for the use of augmentative communication systems', *Language, Speech and Hearing Services in Schools*, XII.

Franklin, J. (1996) 'How Do We Simplify Our Speech With Young Hearing Children?' SENSE, The National Deaf-Blind and Rubella Association.

Hooton, S. (1995) 'Learning disabilities, children and their families', in B. Carter and A. Dearmun (eds) *Child Health Nursing*, Oxford: Blackwell Science.

Hutchfield, K. and Parsons, M. (2003) 'Regular users of children's services: helping to care for children with special needs', *Paediatric Nursing*, 15(2) 36–38.

Jones, O. H. M. (1981) 'Environment and communication: A review', *Special Education Forward Trends*, 8, 22–24.

King, G. A., King, S. M. and Rosenbaum, P. L. (1996) 'Interpersonal aspects of care-giving and client outcomes – a review of the literature', *Ambulatory Child Health*, 2, 151–160.

Kot, A. and Law, J. (1995) 'Intervention with preschool children with specific language impairments; a comparison of two different approaches to treatment', *Child Language Teaching and Therapy*, June, 11(2) 144–162.

Manolson, A. (1992) *It Takes Two to Talk* (3rd edn) Canada: Hanen Centre.

Manolson, A., Ward, B. and Dodington, N. (1995) *You Make the Difference in Helping your Child Learn*, Canada: Hanen Centre.

Marchant, R. and Martyn, M. (1999) *Make it Happen. Communicating with disabled Children: Communication Handbook*, Brighton: Triangle.

Millar, S. and Scott, J. (1998) *Augmentative Communication in practice – an introduction*, University of Edinburgh: Call Centre, Tel: 0131 651 6236.

Millar, S. and Aitken, S. (2003) *Personal Communication Passports: Guidelines for good practice*, University of Edinburgh: Call Centre, Tel: 0131 651 6236.

Morris, J. (1999) *Space For Us. Finding out what disabled children and young people think about their placements*, London: Newham Social Services Department.

Morris, S. E. and Klein, M. D. (1998) *Pre-Feeding Skills*, Tucson, Ariz: Therapy Skill Builders.

Nind, M. and Hewett, D. (1995) *Access to Communication – developing the basics of communication with people with severe learning disabilities through intensive interaction*, London: David Fulton.

Piaget, J. (1975) *The Construction of Reality in the Child*, New York: Ballantyne Books.

Robertson, J. (1970) *Young children in hospital*, London: Tavistock.

Rumble, G. and Larcher, J. (1998) *AAC device review*, Marlow: VOCAtion

Smith, B. (1989) 'Which approach? The education of pupils with SLD', *Mental Handicap* 17, 111–115.

Snow, C. (1977) 'The development of conversation between mothers and babies', *Journal of Child Language* 4.

Stanislawski, N. (1997) 'Lorna's Book' *Talking Sense*, Summer, 26–27.

Tippett, A. (2001) 'All About Me: Documentation for children with special needs', *Paediatric Nursing*, 13(10) December 34–35.

Warner, H. (2000) 'Making the invisible, visible', *Journal of Child Health Care*, 4(3) Autumn, 123–126.

Warner, H. (2001) 'Children with additional needs: The transdisciplinary approach', *Paediatric Nursing*, 13(6) July, 33–36.

Weitzman, E. (1992) *Learning Language and Loving It*, Toronto: Hanen Centre.

Wood, D., Bruner, J. S. and Ross, G. (1976) 'The role of tutoring in problem solving', *Journal of Child Psychology and Psychiatry*, 17, 89–100.

Wong, D. (1999) *The Essentials of Paediatric Nursing*, New York: Mosby.

10 Behaviour, attachment and boundary-setting

Helen K. Warner

Acceptable social behaviour, self-esteem and a sense of security are usually learned within a caring and loving family. However, for some children with a disability, and their families, proactive intervention is necessary, to support the parents to be able to interact appropriately with their child, and begin to come to terms with the reality of their child's care.

Although in previous chapters it has been stated that having a child with a disability is not necessarily a tragedy, in the early days following the birth, and diagnosis, it may well be perceived to be so and a grief response may be triggered for the loss of the perfect child that had been expected and hoped for.

There are many different kinds of loss, but as Pearson (1994) states, they all share common elements, while differing in intensity. When a loss occurs, the overwhelming sense is negative but, however dire, loss also encompasses some positive gains, part of its resolution being the acknowledgement and welcome of these positives.

This chapter will explore how we adapt to loss, and how sometimes parents may need help through this process in order to be able to perceive their child in a realistic way, effectively meet their child's needs, and establish appropriate boundaries.

Often, providing there is support from their spouse and other close relatives, parents may only need informal and minimal professional assistance to help them adapt (Hanson and Hanline 1990). Many mothers feel stressed because they feel unsupported by their partner. Supporting the child's father can enable him to support the mother. Thus the whole family system requires support. In some instances, however, the family may require more formal support systems, such as counselling or psychotherapy, and it has been shown that where family cohesiveness is shaky, mothers are at particular risk for difficulties with parenting and adapting positively to a child with disabilities (Warfield *et al.* 1999).

The grief process

Although we live lives that are constantly changing, we are often ill prepared for loss, especially if the loss is of someone close to us whether by death, divorce or the birth of a less than perfect child. Whatever the loss, a period of grief and mourning will be experienced, and the intensity of feelings is dependent on many things. Worden (1983: 32–34) asserts that although 'the experience of grief is related to the developmental level and conflict issues of the individual involved', the most important determinants fall into seven categories. These are:

- The relationship to the mourner.
- The nature of the attachment.
- The circumstances of the loss.
- Background history.
- Personality.
- Social variables.
- Any concurrent stressors.

Kubler-Ross's (1970) description of grief includes denial, anger, bargaining, depression and acceptance, giving the impression of a neat and tidy sequence, although this is not always the case. Worden (1983), however, in his description of uncomplicated grief discusses the tasks of mourning which are to accept the reality of the loss, experience the pain of grief, adjust to the reality and move on. Therefore grief work involves accepting, adjusting and adapting. Problems can arise at any stage of the grief process and the individual may require help to work them through, although most people are able to cope with grieving on their own. It is important to remember that however well a family may appear to be coping, 'it never gets easy' (McCormack 1992).

Attachment

'Mother love' is not always automatic and many factors influence the way a mother acts towards her baby. These include her reasons for having the baby, experience and competence in childcare, her emotional state, support network and her relationship with the baby's father, together with her social circumstances (Papalia and Olds 1992). Infants also actively influence their carers. Any activity such as crying, smiling, sucking, and looking into the care-giver's eyes, is attachment behaviour. It is the interaction between the adult and infant that determines the attachment behaviour of the infant, and as in any relationship, the partner's responses are crucial. Crittenden and Claussen (2000), building on the work of Bowlby (1982) and Ainsworth's (1971) 'strange situation', suggests that attachment is a theory about developing strategies for predicting and protecting oneself from danger.

Consequently, it is argued that all patterns of attachment are an adaptive response to the context in which they were learned.

Attachment may fail to occur for two broad reasons. The first is that the mother fails to attach to the child due to e.g. loss of the child's 'normality'. The second reason for failure of attachment is that the child fails to attach to the mother, due to the above or due to e.g. autism (autism as an attachment impairment).

If a child has a poor attachment to his primary care-giver, usually the mother, he will have had to 'develop the art of not experiencing his true feelings' (Miller 1987), being too afraid to be himself for fear of being abandoned and losing his mother's love. Children can only experience their feelings if there is someone there who fully accepts, understands and supports them. According to Miller (1987) repressing feelings such as jealousy, envy, anger, loneliness, helplessness and anxiety results in the person's inability to experience them consciously either later in childhood or adulthood. However, those feelings will be stored, and remain in the brain, as information that can be triggered by later events such as a loss and the bereavement process. In these circumstances the bereavement process will be complicated by the repressed feelings, which begin to surface and are accompanied by intense pain and anguish. Miller (1987) describes how, as children we simply could not survive such pain so the feelings are warded off and there is no conscious memory of them, and until these emotions are felt, understood and recognised as legitimate, they will remain repressed. The healing process often means returning to the point where disintegration occurred to enable reintegration to take place, and it is a painful process. There is a need for self-examination, to re-enact or think through the bad times in order to be able to work through them. Early losses, though often dismissed, can therefore have far-reaching consequences and repercussions, and how we deal with later losses therefore depends on how we were reared and on our experiences and perceptions of being mothered/parented (Miller 1987).

Attachment begins and grows as parent and child strengthen their love for each other through touching, smiling and playing. However, the child with developmental delays may not be able to give clear messages of being hungry, tired or over-stimulated. If the parent has difficulty understanding the baby's cues, or the baby does not respond as expected, the 'dance' between them will be interrupted and the parent may need to work much harder to create a secure attachment and help the child to develop a secure sense of self. As the child grows and is dependent on the parent for additional needs as well as the routine holding, feeding and playing each day, the dynamics of love can change between them. Parents may have to switch from the parental role to that of nurse/carer, undertaking tasks e.g. naso-gastric feeds that are not a usual part of parenting. Changing back again to the parental role may then result in role confusion for both the mother and child. However since a positive attachment is so vital to a child's well-being, parents may need to make an extra effort to understand their special child, observing them closely, to learn what each movement or sound he makes may mean, and how he tolerates interactions. As the child grows he will communicate in his own unique way and it is important that parents respond appropriately. Making a child feel as if he is the centre of the universe, and understood, by parents who believe in him no matter what obstacles he may face, is the key to developing a securely attached child. Parents therefore need to be providing a loving, trusting relationship that facilitates attachment; achieves morality in the child by role-modelling concern and empathy for others; enhances cognitive ability by 'scaffolding intellectual experiences' and motivates the child by showing their appreciation of his/her accomplishments (Crittenden and Claussen 2000).

A common initial reaction by mothers however, to a child with disabilities, according to Boone and Hartman (1972), and shown below, is the cyclical response of benevolent overreaction, which results in a cycle of over-protective, permissive parent, and dependent, demanding child.

PARENTS

Guilty, Fearful

CHILD		PARENTS
Insecure	BENEVOLENT	Protective, Permissive
Focus on handicap	OVERREACTION	Indulgent

PARENTS	CHILD
Resentful, Hostile	Dependent, Demanding
Frustrated, Disproportionately	Immature
Angry at times	

This is often a consequence of the parent remaining emotionally distant to the child, due to their own unresolved grief and an insecure attachment. Sometimes feelings are so unbearable that this gets in the way of thinking about practical issues (Shampan 2002). Parents may therefore fear letting the child achieve any new skill, avoid all discipline, and cater to every desire to prevent frustration and a possible tantrum. Unfortunately this will also prevent the child from developing self-control, independence, initiative and self-esteem (Campbell and Glasper 1995). The internal resources of parents, necessary to 'comprehend, digest, and mourn the reality' are taxed to the limit (Reyes-Simpson 2004), requiring them to face their limitations, and to manage despair when there is no hope of change. The capacity of the parent to process the unpalatable truth about their child facilitates the infant's emotional and intellectual development, and enables them to hold on to realistic hopes (Reyes-Simpson 2004).

Children first and foremost

It is important to remember, however, that whatever the child's disability, he still has all the needs of any other child of his age and stage of development that need to be addressed. Children need discipline appropriate to their age and stage of development in order to help them to feel secure. Discipline is not just punishment; it is also about proactively helping children learn what is socially acceptable behaviour, so that they are protected from dangers both within and without, and are encouraged to develop independent thoughts and actions, and relieved of the burden of having to make decisions they are not yet equipped to make (Campbell and Glasper 1995). This is best achieved in a positive way by setting limits on the child's behaviour and consistently enforcing them so that the child can learn what his limitations are and what is expected of him, secure in the knowledge that his adult carers are in control. Jenner (1999) describes the Attention Rule and Child Centred Behaviours as an effective way to teach children what is acceptable (see below):

THE ATTENTION RULE

- **Praise every sociable action of your child with enthusiasm**
- **Praise your child frequently just for being themselves**

- **Ignore 99 per cent of minor naughty behaviours**

- **Punish only physically dangerous behaviours, emotionally hurtful actions or words and unsafe destructiveness**

- **Use lots of child centred behaviours**

(from Jenner (1999) *The Parent/Child Game*, London: Bloomsbury)

Child centred behaviours

Attends

- Describing out loud to your child, with warmth and enthusiasm, what they are doing (as long as you approve, of course).

    E.g. 1)   'Oh! You've made a really *tasty* sandwich!'
    2)   'You've chosen the red paints to do that *lovely* apple!'

- Commenting positively on how your child looks.

    E.g. 1)   'You look *great* in that tee-shirt!'
    2)   'Your hair looks really cool with that gel on!'

- Noticing out loud, in a positive way, your child's mood.

    E.g. 1)   'You're concentrating so hard.'
    2)   'You seem to have lots of energy today.'

Praises

- Clearly expressing your approval and delight towards your child.

    E.g. 1)   'You're so clever!'
       2)   'You're such fun to be with!'

- Reacting to your child's behaviour, play and conversation warmly and enthusiastically.

    E.g. 1)   'Well done! That's a great effort!'
       2)   'Fabulous! What a good joke!'

Smiles

- Making eye contact with your child and smiling right into their eyes in a loving and friendly way.

    E.g. 1)   Giving a warm, spontaneous smile *to* your child.
       2)   Laughing or giggling *with* your child

Imitation

- Copying your child's actions or words so that they can tell you are interested in them.

    E.g. 1)   'OK, so you'd like honey on your cereal, not sugar.'
       2)   'You're going to build a bridge,' when they say, 'I'm going to make a bridge.'

- Imitating with genuine enthusiasm, any noises your child might make when playing.

    E.g. 1)   'Vroom, vroom,' when playing cars.
       2)   'Maaa, maaa,' when playing farms.

Ask to play

- Asking your child what they would like you to play with them.

    E.g. 1)   'What game would you like me to play with you now?'
       2)   'You can choose what to play and then tell me what I should do.'

- Asking your child what they would like you to do.

    E.g. 1)   'What would you like me to do next?'
       2)   'Tell me what you want me to do right now.'

- Allowing your child to tell you that they would like you to sit and watch them, and complying with their wishes.
- Encouraging your child to lead the activities or game.

Ignore minor naughtiness

● Turn your head away, look bored and keep silent.

E.g. 1) Noticeably ignore your child when they are doing something that's naughty in a minor and non-dangerous way.

2) Make no comment but look away, half-turning your shoulder or body from them, only returning your attention when your child's behaviour is once more acceptable.

Positive touches

● Give your child a warm, affectionate hug, kiss, pat or stroke.

E.g. 1) These must be touches that the child welcomes and enjoys

2) The hugs, kisses, squeezes and strokes which you give your child must always be appropriate to their stage of development.

(from Jenner, S. (1999) *The Parent/Child Game*, London: Bloomsbury)

Psychological development

The capacity to deal with uncertainty and loss is determined by the individual's internal state, skill, and the support and encouragement which they receive (Broome 1990). Our internal state, or what we are like, according to Winnicott (1986) depends on where we have arrived in our emotional development. Winnicott (1986) argues that if parenting is 'good enough' the mother enables her baby to experience omnipotence, an awareness that the child only has to reach out for whatever is wanted and it is there for the taking. Babies need to experience this all-powerful feeling before they lose it in the process of learning about the reality principle. Thus disillusionment can only occur on the basis of illusion, and 'if we have been happy, we can bear distress' argues Winnicott (1986: 47). The implication is that if we have not experienced happiness, then it is much more difficult to bear distress.

Erikson's theory of psychological development, essentially states the same thing but in a different way. According to Erikson (1963), all human beings pass through eight stages, and each stage has to be worked through before embarking on the following stage. Should any stage not be fully resolved, the ability to move on to the next is limited, so inhibiting development. However, something that is not resolved in an individual's development may, to some extent, be completed at a later date.

The first stage of Erikson's theory is that infants learn trust or mistrust. If there is a secure attachment between a mother and her baby the baby will learn to trust that his/her needs will be met. This is the 'good enough' parenting described by Winnicott (1986), which is demonstrated by the mother's attentiveness and responsiveness to the baby. If, however, the parenting is inadequate, it may be experienced as rejecting, and unreliable, resulting in the infant feeling that there is something wrong with him, and which makes him a bad person for having all these needs to be met, argues Winnicott (1986). The child becomes afraid to be himself, controlling himself so that his behaviour becomes what he perceives is expected of him; for example, in the Romanian Orphanages in the 1980s, children were shown to lie quietly in their cots because they had learned that crying did not get them the attention they needed.

The writer has attempted to show how early experiences and perceptions of their own parenting will affect the way parents deal with the loss of their 'perfect' child. Cultural beliefs and religion are also important factors and will influence the family's reactions to a child with disability, and may include guilt and self-blame. It will therefore be important not to make any assumptions but to allow parents to express themselves, acknowledging and accepting what they are saying. When parents grieve for the loss of the child they had hoped and planned for, the bereavement process itself may inhibit bonding with the child and also the ability to bond, the adults being emotionally preoccupied with their own issues with no space left to be able to look to the child's emotional needs.

Models of adaptation

The process that follows the diagnosis of a child with disability and which focuses on a series of stages has been explained by models of adaptation as shown in Table 10.1.

Implications for nurses

During the parental period of adjustment, four possible reactions to the child will influence the child's own eventual response to their disability, according to Campbell and Glasper (1995), and these include over-protection, rejection, denial and gradual acceptance.

Over-protection is such a common parental reaction that it is important for nurses to be able to recognise when it is occurring so that counselling may be offered to enable the parent to have more realistic expectations of their child by changing their perceptions, which in turn will have a positive effect on their relationship with the child. This response is one that responds well to early intervention and counselling may be carried out by a health professional, already known to the family, and who has training in the use of counselling skills or by a trained counsellor or psychologist. However, this is a sensitive area and there remains a certain stigma to the use of counselling. It will be important to reassure the family that having counselling is not a sign of failure but instead a positive and proactive measure to get the emotional support they require so that their relationship with their child may be enhanced. It is therefore also important that nurses are able to identify where the family is in terms of the grieving process so that appropriate support can

Table 10.1 Models of adaptation to diagnosis of disability

Hornby (1994)		Miller et al (1994)	
Stage	Associated emotion	Stage	Associated emotion/ behaviour
Shock	Confusion Numbness	Surviving	Shock, fatigue, physical symptoms fragility and vulnerability. Grief, sadness, depression, chaos and confusion, guilt
Denial	Disbelief Protest		Self-absorption, shame, embarrassment Resentment and envy, unconscious denial
Anger	Blame Guilt	Searching	Begins while still surviving Quest for diagnosis, contact with other families, gaining competence and control, forced self-development, Acknowledging that you are a different person because you have a child with special needs
Sadness	Despair Grief		
Detachment	Emptiness Meaninglessness		
Reorganisation	Realism Hope	Settling in	Realisation there are no quick cures and no answers to some questions. Become aware of regular progress in child's development. Get on with the rest of your life. New knowledge and skills
Adaptation	Reconciliation Coming to terms		Develop a network of people. Increased flexibility and adaptability
		Separating	Giving some control over to child and others. Pride in child's achievements.

Source: adapted from Barr (1997).

be offered if they appear to be stuck or resistant to change. Full acceptance of how the family members may be feeling is vital, remembering that we feel what we feel, and there are no rights or wrongs.

Acknowledgement of whatever the family is feeling and allowing them the space to talk things through is the first step in helping them come to terms with their reality. This can be difficult when what the family is feeling is anger, which is another common reaction, and one that may be targeted at the health professionals. Smith (1992) asserts that nurses cannot be blamed if they fear having to deal with parents who are struggling with their violent emotions. It will, however, be important to remember that the anger is not intended to be personally critical, even though the family may be critical of

nursing or medical care, but part of the grieving process. The gradual acceptance of their child's difficulties, will enable parents to place necessary and
realistic restrictions on the child, encourage self-care activities, and promote
reasonable physical and social abilities (Campbell and Glasper 1995).

The difficulties for parents when their child is in hospital will be compounded when they are faced with nurses who may have little experience of
caring for a child with a disability. The extra effort parents have to make to
bond with and care for their child, perhaps need to be reflected in the extra
effort required by nurses to care for both parent and child when in hospital.
It may also be difficult for the children themselves who may attempt to evoke
the response they are used to and fail. It is therefore important that nurses
respond positively to the signals the child is giving, and recognise the child's
need to test the boundaries. If nurses have their own boundaries and thus
model boundary-setting for parents, in a sensisitive way, parents may be
helped to recognise the need to help their child behave in more acceptable
and appropriate ways. However there is a danger of the nurse/counsellor
appearing so capable that the parent(s) feels even more inadequate. Thus
enormous sensitivity must be demonstrated by the nurse.

Being able to recognise behaviours in the child which may suggest poor
attachment will help nurses to ensure that families receive appropriate support when they need it. Children who have poor attachment strategies, in a
similar way to parents preoccupied by their grief, may be so preoccupied by
their attempts to get the attention they need that they tend not to explore
their environment, react rather than interact and may cause their carers to
respond negatively to them. They may be delayed in their development,
withdrawn and unresponsive. However, for the child with disabilities, who is
at greater risk of attachment difficulties than a typical child, and who may
already be delayed in their development, withdrawn and unresponsive due to
their disability, it may be easier to identify any attachment difficulties from
the way in which they are parented:

- Persistent ambivalent or negative feelings towards the child.
- Appears indifferent to the child, and relates to the child in an impersonal way.
- Sees child as unattractive.
- Develops inappropriate responses to the infant's needs e.g. under- or over-feeding, over-stimulating or under-stimulating, forcing or refusing eye contact, bouncing or tickling infant when the infant is tired.
- Cannot discriminate between infant's signals for hunger, comfort, rest, body contact.
- Believes the infant is judging him/her and does not love him/her.
- Develops paradoxical attitudes and behaviours towards the infant.

(adapted from Campbell and Glasper, 1995)

References

Ainsworth, M. D. S., Bell, S. M. and Stayton, D. J. (1971) 'Individual differences in Strange Situation behaviour of one-year-olds', in H. R. Schaffer (ed.), *The Origin of Human Social Relations*, London: Academic Press.

Barr, O. (1997) 'Interventions in a family context', in B. Gates (ed.) *Learning Disabilities*, (3rd edn) London: Churchill Livingstone.

Boone, D. R. and Hartman, B. H. (1972) 'The Benevolent Overreaction', *Clinical Pediatrics* 11(5) 268–271.

Bowlby, J. (1971) *Attachment and Loss*, Harmondsworth: Penguin.

Bowlby, J. (1982) *Attachment* (vol. 1), New York: Basic Books.

Broome, A. (1990) 'Working for change', *Nursing Times*, 86(19) 30–31.

Campbell, S. and Glasper, E. A. (1995) *Whaley and Wong's Children's Nursing*, London: Mosby.

Crittenden, P. and Claussen, A. (2000) *The Organization of Attachment Relationships: Maturation, Culture and Context*, New York: Cambridge University Press.

Erikson, E. (1963) *Childhood and Society*, Harmondsworth: Penguin.

Hanson, M. J. and Hanline, M. F. (1990) 'Parenting a child with a disability: A longitudinal study of parental stress and adaptation', *Journal of Early Intervention* 14, 234–248.

Hornby, G. (1994) *Counselling in child disability. Skills for working with parents*, London: Chapman and Hall.

Jacobs, M. (1988) *Psychodynamic Counselling in Action*, London: Sage.

Jenner, S. (1999) *The Parent/Child Game*, London: Bloomsbury.

Kubler-Ross, E. (1970) *On Death and Dying*, London: Routledge.

McCormack, M. (1992) *Special Children, Special Needs. Families talk about living with mental handicap*, London: Thorsons.

Miller, A. (1987) *The Drama of Being a Child*, London: Virage Press.

Miller, N. B., Burmester, S., Callahan, D. G., Dieterle, J. and Niedermeyer, S. (1994) *Nobody's perfect*, Baltimore: Paul H. Brookes.

Papalia, D. and Olds, W. (1992) *Human Development*, (5th edn) New York: McGraw-Hill.

Pearson, A. (1994) *Growing through Grief and Loss*, London: HarperCollins.

Reyes-Simpson, E. (2004) 'When there is too much to take in: some factors that restrict the capacity to think', chapter 9 in D. Simpson and L. Miller (eds) *Unexpected Gains: Psychotherapy with people with Learning Disabilities*, London: Karnac Books.

Shampan, L. (2002) *Parents Have Needs Too! The role of counselling services for children with special needs and disabilities*, Greenford: 3Cs Counselling Service.

Smith, P. (1992) *The Emotional Labour of Nursing*, London: Macmillan.

Warfield, M., Krauss, M., Hauser-Cram, P., Upshur, C. and Shonkoff, J. (1999) 'Adaptation during early childhood among mothers of children with disabilities', *Developmental and Behavioural Pediatrics*, 20(1) February, 9–16.

Winnicott, D. W. (1986) *Home is where we Start From – Essays by a Psychoanalyst*, Harmondsworth: Penguin.

Worden, W. J. (1983) *Grief Counselling and Grief Therapy*, London: Routledge.

Further reading

Ainsworth, M. and Eichberg, C. (1991) 'Effects on infant-mother attachment of mothers' unresolved loss of an Attachment Figure', in P. Marris, J. Stevenson-Hinde and C. Parkes (eds) *Attachment Across the Life-Cycle*, New York: Routledge, pp. 160–183.

Faber, A. and Mazlish, E. (2001) *How to Talk so Kids will Listen and Listen so Kids will Talk*, London: Piccadilly Press.

Siegal, D. J. (1999) *The Developing Mind: Toward a Neurobiology of Interpersonal Experience*, Sussex: Guilford Press.

Train, A. (2000) *Children Behaving Badly*, London: Souvenir Press.

11 Pain assessment in the acute setting

Helen K. Warner

A book regarding the care of children with disabilities, in the acute setting, would be incomplete without a chapter on pain and its assessment. Schecter (1989) asserted that children's pain management is generally less effective than that of adults, and nine years later, McGrath *et al.* (1998) stated that children, who have a neurological or cognitive impairment, are at particular risk of having their pain underestimated and under-treated.

Pain management for children is an area that has received little attention in the literature until recent years, and particularly for those children who have a cognitive impairment or developmental delay, and yet this group of children seem to have an increased risk of pain, both from the activities of daily living as well as from invasive procedures (Oberlander *et al.* 1999). Stallard *et al.* (2001) assert that failure to identify and treat pain causes unnecessary suffering and distress to children and increased parental and family stress, while at the same time they found that the experience of pain was common, although active pain relief is not. In extreme cases the inability to recognise signs of pain can lead to fatality (Donovan 1997). However, Lebeer (1992) found that the assessment of pain is *ad hoc*, based mainly on medical and nursing intuition, together with informal family reports.

This chapter will consider the increased sources of pain for this group of children, compared to children in general, as well as a discussion of the altered pain experience, which is so relevant for this group of children. An examination of the knowledge required to assess and manage their pain will be attempted and a short discussion of possible reasons why pain and discomfort in children with more severe learning disabilities may be overlooked and inadequately treated. There will be a discussion about altered pain experiences and tactile defensiveness, ending with a list of suggested activities to encourage and enable integration of the senses to take place and the defensiveness overcome.

Sources of pain

Hunt *et al*. (2003) describe four main categories of pain:

- Pain associated with altered gut motility e.g. gastro-oesophageal reflux, wind and constipation.
- Pain associated with muscle spasm, dislocated hips, joint and back pain.
- Pain generally associated with a lack of mobility such as pressure sores.
- Coincidental pains e.g. toothache and earache and pain related to badly fitting aids and equipment such as splints and casts used to prevent contractures.

Even communication, although not typically perceived to be painful has been reported as a source of discomfort, by adolescents using mechanical devices (Oberlander *et al*. 1999). For those who are unable to swallow and who rely on gastrostomy tubes or other forms of enteral nutrition, other sources of pain may be feelings of gastric distention, or pulling on the site and skin breakdown. This last, or fifth, category of pain includes all invasive procedures including surgery to manage the consequences of the underlying condition e.g. surgical intervention for high muscle tone/spasticity or by the surgical implantation of an intrathecal baclofen pump.

Altered pain experiences

Biersdorff (1994) suggests that children with neurological impairments have an altered pain experience relating to pain insensitivity and indifference. Pain insensitivity is the inability to distinguish between sharp and blunt sensations, or hot and cold due to problems in the sensory neurones of the peripheral or central nervous system. On the other hand pain indifference is attributed to those who have difficulty in evaluating sensations so that although they can feel the sharpness of a needle, they do not find it painful. Biersdorff (1994) concluded that carers need to increase their vigilance when caring for those with a high pain threshold and that for reasons of safety, the children/young people themselves require training to recognise dangerous situations and to be alert to possible sources of injuries such as cuts and burns.

Sensory integration theory

If we look at sensory integration theory, first described by an occupational therapist 30–40 years ago (Ayres 1998), it may help to explain the altered pain perceptions/experiences of some children. Until about age seven, Ayres (1998) argues that the brain is primarily a sensory processing machine and young children are in the sensory-motor stage of development. Our senses inform us about the physical condition of our bodies, and the environment around us, and include an additional sense that detects the pull of gravity and our bodily movements in relation to the earth (ibid.). Information taken in through our senses is organised or integrated in our brain to enable us to make sense of the world and adapt our responses to it. In this way our brain uses sensations to direct our minds and bodies. The pages of this book, however, are not sufficient to go into sensory integration theory in great depth, but it must be said that for children who experience developmental delays it would not be surprising if they did not also experience delays in the development of their sensory system and the integration of their senses. Sensory Integrative therapy has been shown to be effective for many children with learning and behaviour problems and is usually carried out by an occupational therapist or physiotherapist specifically trained to do so (ibid.). Integration of the senses occurs in the pre-conscious brain and is closely linked with the parts of the brain responsible for the emotions i.e. the limbic system and the amygdala. There is, therefore, a relationship between the integration of the senses and our behaviour. According to sensory integration theory, none of us organises or integrates sensations perfectly although 'happy productive, well-coordinated people may come the closest to perfect sensory integration' (ibid.).

Poor sensory integration, on the other hand, will interfere with every aspect of life, causing more difficulties and effort and less success and satisfaction (Ayres 1998). Only trained observers can detect the subtle differences between behaviour based on good sensory integration and that based on poor integration. It is not something that can be measured, and only through observation and sensory integration diagnostic tests is it possible to try and judge how a child's brain is functioning. A delay in language development is common and an early clue that all is not well in the brain. Some children cannot organise sensations from their skin e.g. they may become anxious or angry when touched or if people stand close to them. For others, sometimes light or noise will cause irritation and distraction and close observation will detect the irritation in the child's face. Indeed, Ayres asserted that poor sensory integration is responsible for much of the hyperactivity that we commonly see in children today.

The tactile system

Tactile defensiveness is a subtle yet serious neural disorder and is frequently seen in children with learning disabilities, minimal brain dysfunction and more serious conditions (Ayres 1998). Sensory messages are received through the skin, which is the largest sensory organ of the body. It receives some of our most basic sensory information – touch (location, identifying things without vision), pressure (soft, firm, ticklish), pain (danger?), and temperature (hot/cold). The development of this primitive system is necessary before higher level, (cortical) skills appear, and develop normally i.e. motor planning and coordination.

The tactile system consists of two parts. The protective system, which is responsible for the body automatically withdrawing or defending itself from touch that is interpreted as harmful, leading to a flight or fight response. The second part of this system is the discriminative system, and this provides the brain with precise information regarding size, shape and texture of objects in the environment. It tells us where we're being touched and what is touching us.

The balance of these systems is essential if the tactile system is to work properly. If the protective system is overloaded, the discriminative system cannot work well and this can lead to over-sensitivity (hyper-responsiveness) or under-sensitivity (hypo-responsiveness). Treatment aims to balance these two nerve pathways and allow the discriminative pathway to work more freely, letting the child's skills develop, reducing their distractability and increasing concentration.

Hyper-responsiveness

These children will notice and be bothered by things that most of us will not even notice:

- Dislike being cuddled, but will seek out touch on their own terms – initiated and controlled by them.
- Dislike being close to people, avoid crowds, get upset if someone unexpectedly bumps or brushes against them.
- Aggressive in their interaction with others.
- Find certain types of clothes irritating, be very sensitive to certain textures, labels and new clothes.
- Respond badly to clothes/nappy being changed.
- OVER-SENSITIVE TO PAIN AND PHYSICAL HURT.
- Greater sensitivity than normal to having hair cut/washed, teeth brushed, nails cut.
- Avoid walking barefoot on grass/sand.
- Walk on toes, dislike wearing socks and shoes, or prefer to always wear socks and shoes.
- Avoid using the palms of hands.
- Avoid messy play – hate dirty hands/feet.
- Oversensitive/aversion to food textures especially soft foods.
- Seem to be over-emotional – irritable, withdrawn, angry.
- Poor attention because they are over alert to being touched.
- Bonding difficulties due to avoidance of touch/cuddles by others.

This may often lead to the FLIGHT/FRIGHT/FIGHT RESPONSES:

FLIGHT: verbal/non-verbal avoidance, loners, class clowns, restless/changes position/leaves room frequently.

FRIGHT: shy/reluctant to communicate, problems with early childhood bonding, decreased attention due to over awareness of others.

FIGHT: problem-child, negative/resistant behaviour, physically/verbally aggressive, agitated when people get close to them but often inappropriately close to others.

Hypo-responsiveness

These children may come across as touch 'hungry':

● Under-awareness of being touched.
● May appear passive and inactive.
● DECREASED SENSITIVITY TO PHYSICAL PAIN.
● May touch others inappropriately and be unaware of the intensity of their touch/pressure.
● Difficulty manipulating toys.
● Difficulty recognising and manipulating objects without vision.

Thus problems with sensory processing can result in altered pain experiences, and often the child will also be emotionally insecure (Ayres 1998), the disorder in the tactile system also making the emotions easily upset.

Gate-control theory of pain

This theory suggests that pain perception can be influenced by psychosocial factors so that if these are positive the 'gate' will be closed, so that less pain is perceived. However if the factors are negative the 'gate' will be opened, making the pain feel worse (Melzack and Wall 1988). The 'gate' in question is a hypothetical 'gate' situated in the dorsal column of the spinal cord through which the pain impulses must pass on their way to the brain. It may be argued that someone with a severe learning disability may feel less pain because they do not understand the potential consequence of the pain and therefore do not become anxious about it. On the other hand it may be argued that less understanding and a lack of control may lead to increased tension and anxiety and consequently more pain. Consequently when children are admitted to hospital, and may experience a lack of understanding, feelings of isolation and loss of their familiar routine and familiar family members around them, they may experience enhanced pain.

Assessment of pain

Freedom from pain is a basic human right limited only by our knowledge to achieve it (Liebeskind and Melzack 1988). Defining pain is very difficult, as it is a subjective feeling, but McCaffrey's (1994) definition is generally accepted, that 'pain is what the person experiencing it says it is'. By definition then, those children who cannot easily communicate when or where they have pain or the intensity of the pain are faced with an immediate problem. Tesler and colleagues (1989) compiled a list of 129 words used by children to describe the intensity of their pain, including words to describe the pain sensation e.g. 'throbbing' or 'gnawing', as well as the emotional aspect e.g. 'fearful' or 'exhausting'. Words can also describe the individual's evaluation of their pain e.g. 'annoying' or 'unbearable' and whether it is 'constant' or 'rhythmic'.

Children who are unable to communicate verbally are clearly at a disadvantage when it comes to expressing their pain. Carter and colleagues (2002), however, showed that even though they may have a limited repertoire of behaviours available to them, children are able to express pain. In less severe cases, as Donovan (1997) suggests, signs or pictures can be used e.g. there are Makaton signs for 'How are you?' 'pain,' 'ill', and 'sick'. Also photographs showing a range of facial expressions from 'pain-free' to 'severe pain' can be used for the self-reporting of pain (Beyer 1989), and the location of pain can be indicated using body drawings or models. It is recommended that pain assessment includes the use of a validated pain assessment tool (RCN 2002). However, Fanurik *et al.* (1998) argued that nurses tend to over-estimate the abilities of children with a cognitive impairment to use a rating scale, and suggested the importance of children being asked to demonstrate their ability to understand and use such a scale before it is used to assess their pain.

Alternatively nurses can use their observation skills to recognise pain behaviours. Fordyce (1976) described four groups of non-verbal pain behaviours (see Table 11.1).

It was proposed by Anand and Craig (1996) that the behavioural changes caused by pain in non-verbal children should be recognised as a form of self-report that would optimise pain management. However, children with neurological impairments do not necessarily display 'typical' pain behaviours such as moaning or facial expressions that reflect their pain and may show idiosyncratic behaviours that are pain related (McGrath *et al.* 1998; Breau *et al.* 2000).

Bearing in mind the above studies that reiterate the need to involve parents, Hunt and colleagues (2003) assert that parents and professionals have traditionally thought it important to 'know the child' well, in order to be able to ascertain how he reacts to pain. Hunt *et al.* (2004), however, found that when using the paediatric pain profile, a behaviour rating scale generated by Hunt (2001) in a hospital setting, the extent of the clinician's familiarity with the child did not appear to significantly affect the results, and they suggested that the use of a behaviour rating scale may reduce the subjectivity of the judgement made.

Table 11.1 Pain behaviour

Non-language	Crying
	Screaming
	Sighing
	Moaning
Body posturing	Grimacing
	Clenched teeth
	Shutting eyes
	Clenched fists
	Limping
	Flinching and gesturing
	Head in hands
	Muscle tension
	Protective actions i.e. guarding or bracing the injured site
Functional limitation	Not able to work/play
	Reduced range of movement
	Lying or sitting down for long periods
Pain-reducing behaviour	Rubbing injured part
	Approaching staff
	Avoiding excessive sensory stimulation e.g. sounds and lights

Source: adapted from Fordyce (1976).

Paediatric Pain Profile (PPP)

Hunt's (2001) Paediatric Pain Profile consists of three sets of recordings as follows:

- A retrospective rating made by the parent of the child's behaviour when the child is at his/her best.
- Retrospective ratings of the child's behaviour during any current or recurring pain.
- Future/prospective ratings

Hunt *et al.* (2004) suggest that the assessments are completed during discussion between the parent, and a clinician who regularly works with the family. In this way it is suggested that screening is provided for the child's current state, which, at the same time provides a reference for future assessments and encouragement of a dialogue between parent and professional about the child's current pain difficulties. The PPP (Table 11.2) also provides a tool to monitor the impact of therapeutic interventions. The profile is intended to be parent-held and jointly maintained by the parents and professionals involved in their child's care. The profile is also intended to accompany the child wherever he goes e.g. GP, hospital, school, and respite care. Should the child already have a personal communication passport (see Chapter 9), the writer would suggest that this information is incorporated into the

Table 11.2 The 20-item Paediatric Pain Profile

During the last . . . (first name)	Not at all	A little	Quite a lot	A great deal	Unable to assess
1 Was cheerful					
2 Was sociable or responsive					
3 Withdrawn or depressed					
4 Cried/moaned/groaned/screamed or whimpered					
5 Hard to console/comfort					
6 Bit self or banged head					
7 Reluctant to eat/difficult to feed (includes nasogastric and gastrostomy feeding)					
8 Disturbed sleep					
9 Grimaced/screwed up face/screwed up eyes					
10 Frowned/had furrowed brow/looked worried					
11 Looked frightened (eyes wide open)					
12 Ground teeth or made mouthing movements					
13 Restless/agitated or distressed					
14 Tense/stiffened or spasmed					
15 Flexed inwards or drew legs up towards chest					
16 Tended to touch/rub particular areas					
17 Resisted being moved					
18 Pulled away or flinched when touched					
19 Twisted and turned/tossed head/ writhed or arched back					
20 Involuntary or stereotypical movements/was jumpy or had seizures					

Source: adapted from Hunt *et al.* (2004).

existing document, to avoid confusion, and to ensure that *all* of the child's needs can be met appropriately.

Knowledge required to assess pain

Hunt and colleagues (2003) describe three forms of knowledge that are important when assessing and managing pain in this population of children. These are:

- Knowing the child and having the ability to recognise changes in their behaviour in different contexts.
- Familiarity with the population and the ability to recognise similarities and differences between children.
- Knowing the 'science'.

Hunt and colleagues (2003) demonstrated that each of these forms of knowledge is held by different parties to the child's care, and only in a minority of cases does one person hold all three types of knowledge. This may be one explanation of why pain and discomfort in this population of children may be overlooked and inadequately treated. Another explanation is that the attitudes and beliefs of health professionals adversely affect the recognition and management of pain. Watt-Watson (1987) and Vortherms and colleagues (1992), cited by Oberlander and colleagues (1999), showed that incorrect assumptions about the quality and quantity of pain as well as the risks of addiction have resulted in widespread under-treatment of pain in children and although this has not specifically been demonstrated for children with neurological impairment it seems likely that it would also apply to them. The view that attitudes of some health professionals are less than desirable is supported by Carter and colleagues (2002), who showed that while parents have an intimate knowledge of their child's usual non-pain state, they often feel isolated and under-used by professionals in relation to pain management. Parents were also found to feel that their child had learnt to live with significant levels of acute and chronic pain due to less than optimal pain management.

Conclusion

It seems clear from the above that the best way of managing children's pain is to work collaboratively with parents and families so that there is a sharing and understanding of the information required. Previous chapters have shown how different professionals and experts, including parents, all have a small piece of the picture and only when there is a coming together of all involved can the whole picture be seen and understood. Can it be any different when it comes to pain? There is increasing evidence that parents are best placed and adept at assessing behavioural changes that suggest their child is in pain (Callery 1997; McGrath *et al.* 1998).

The Paediatric Pain Profile (Hunt 2001, www.ppp.co.uk) provides a tool for assessing pain in children with severe to profound neurological disabilities and the opportunity for collaboration between parents and professionals to optimise the quality of the assessment, which with continuing use, may show a pattern of behaviours unique to the individual. However, to manage pain appropriately it is not enough to simply react to pain behaviours observed in the child, but to proactively look, listen and feel for them (Hunt *et al.* 2003). The child's change in tone can also be felt through kinaesthetic sensations so that it is important not to forget this source of knowing in addition to 'looking' and 'listening'.

Finally access to the 'science' is of equal importance and it may be that nursing staff will require further training in this area, and, in addition, support from the pain management team, particularly when managing complex postoperative regimes (Oberlander *et al.* 1999).

Furthermore it is important to understand the effects of the child's pain on the parents' lives as well as the child him/herself. Hunt and colleagues (2003) remind us that that understanding alone can help to ease parental distress. Similarly understanding that parental anxiety may also affect the child's pain (McGrath and McAlpine 1993) may help to motivate nurses to attempt to alleviate parental anxiety. Understanding the pain experience in this way and the meaning that experience has for the individual can also be the motivator needed to find ways to alleviate the child's distress. Finally, as Savins (2002) reminds us, it is difficult for anyone to witness children in pain and professionals themselves require support to deal with their fears, so that they are able to respond appropriately and creatively to children's pain.

Suggested activities for tactile defensiveness

It is important to remember never to forcefully impose tactile stimulation on a child with a tactile system problem, but to respect their cues of when to stop. Encourage them to actively explore and watch carefully for 'overload'. Wherever possible, play with as much skin exposed as possible, e.g. shoes and socks off! Avoid light, ticklish touch and use firm and consistent pressure. Avoid irritation situations until the problem is alleviated, as this will just elicit negative reactions and further avoidance.

- Play with toys and materials that vary in texture (soft, hard, rough, smooth, pliable, light, heavy).
- Play with sand – wet or dry.
- Water play – different temperatures, contrasting hot (not too hot!) and cold, with or without bubbles, spraying, dripping, splashing etc.
- Give a good firm rub with a towel.
- Use firm massage on hands and feet, using circular movements.
- Hide objects in different textures – sand, pasta, lentils, polystyrene pieces.
- Make a tactile collage using a variety of fabrics etc.
- Use play-dough – pinching, kneading, rolling out with the hands, twisting.
- Play with rings and bracelets to increase awareness of hands and individual fingers.
- Use shaving foam, spray cream or packet whipped pudding to play with, bury hands into, spread it out, pull it together.
- Roll/crawl/jump on textured material – furry mats, bubble wrap, carpet.
- Wrap firmly in a sheet or blanket and unroll by pulling one end.
- Crawl through tight spaces.
- Heavy work activities like push/pull games and jumping games.
- Rough and tumble games (be careful not to 'overload').
- Action rhymes and songs involving parts of the body.
- Use food with different textures.
- Dressing is also a great activity to encourage tactile processing.

References

Anand, K. J. S. and Craig, K. D. (1996) 'New perspectives on the definition of pain', *Pain* 67: 3–6.

Ayres, A. J. (1998) *Sensory Integration and the Child* (13th edn) Western Psychological Services.

Beyer, J. (1989) 'The oucher: a pain intensity scale for children', in S. Funk (ed.) *Management of Pain, Fatigue and Nausea*, New York: Springer.

Biersdorff, K. K. (1994) 'Incidence of significantly altered pain experience among individuals with developmental disabilities', *American Journal of Mental Retardation*, 98(5) 619–631.

Breau, L. M., McGrath, P. J., Camfield, C., Rosmus, C. and Finley, G. A. (2000) 'Preliminary validation of an observational pain checklist for persons with cognitive impairments and inability to communicate verbally', *Developmental Medicine and Child Neurology*, 42(9) 609–616.

Callery, P. (1997) 'Maternal Knowledge and professional knowledge: co-operation and conflict in the care of sick children', *International Journal of Nursing Studies*, 34(1) 27–34.

Carter, B., McArthur, E. and Cunliffe, M. (2002) 'Dealing with uncertainty: parental assessment of pain in their children with profound special needs', *Journal of Advanced Nursing*, 38(5) 449–457.

Davies, D. Evans, L. (2001) 'Assessing Pain in People with Profound Learning Disability', *British Journal Nursing* 10.8: 481–552.

Donovan, J. (1997) 'Pain Signals', *Nursing Times*, November 5(93) 45, 60–62.

Fanurik, D., Koh, J. L., Harrison, R. D., Conrad, T. M. and Tomerlin, C. (1998) 'Pain Assessment in Children with Cognitive Impairment', *Clinical Nursing Research*, 7(2) May 1998, 103–124.

Fordyce, W. (1976) *Behavioural Methods for Chronic Pain and Illness*, St Louis, Miss.: Mosby.

Hunt, A. M. (2001) 'Towards an understanding of pain in the child with severe neurological impairment. Development of a behaviour rating scale for assessing pain', unpublished Ph.D. Thesis, University of Manchester.

Hunt, A. M., Mastroyannopoulou, K., Goldman, A. and Seers, K. (2003) 'Not Knowing – the problem of pain in children with severe neurological impairment', *International Journal of Nursing Studies* 40, 171–183.

Hunt, A., Goldman, A., Seers, K., Mastroyannopoulou, K., Moffat, V., Oulton, K. and Brady, M. (2004) 'Clinical Validation of the Paediatric Pain Profile', *Developmental Medicine and Child Neurology* 46, 9–18.

Lebeer, J. (1992) 'Families with a handicapped child: dealing with pain', in A. Kaplun (ed.) *Health Promotion and Chronic Illness. Discovering a New Quality of Health*, WHO Regional Publications Series, No 44.

Liebeskind, J. C. and Melzack, R. (1988) 'The International Pain Foundation: Meeting the need for education in pain management', *Journal of Pain and Symptom Management* 3(3) 131–134.

McCaffrey, M. (1994) *Pain: Clinical Manual for Nursing Practice*, London: Mosby.

McGrath, P. and McAlpine, L. (1993) 'Psychologic perspectives on paediatric pain', *The Journal of Paediatrics*, 122(5) 2.

McGrath, P. J., Rosmus, C., Canfield, C., Campbell, M. A. and Hennidar, A. (1998) 'Behaviours caregivers use to determine pain in non-verbal, cognitively impaired individuals', *Developmental Medicine and Child Neurology*, 40, 340–343.

Melzack, P. and Wall, P. (1988) *The Challenge of Pain*, London: Penguin.

Oberlander, T. F., O'Donnell, M. E. and Montgomery, C. J. (1999) 'Pain in Children with Significant Neurological Impairment', *Developmental and Behavioural Pediatrics* 20(4) 235–243.

Royal College of Nursing (1999) *The recognition and assessment of acute pain in Children: recommendations*, London: RCN.

Savins, C. (2002) 'Therapeutic work with children in pain' *Paediatric Nursing*, 14(5) June, 14–16.

Schecter, N. L. (1989) 'The under-treatment of pain in children: an overview' *Pediatric Clinics of North America*, 36(4) 781–793.

Stallard P., Williams L., Lenton S. and Velleman, R. (2001) 'Pain in cognitively impaired, Non-communicating children, *Archives of Disease in Childhood* 85, 460–462.

Tesler, M. (1989) 'Children's words for pain', in S. Funk (ed.) *Management of Pain, Fatigue and Nausea*, New York: Springer.

12 Managing difficult behaviour in the acute setting

Catherine Bernal

Case scenario

Jack is 7 years old. He has autism and also an under-functioning thyroid gland for which he takes thyroxine medication. Jack has a very limited diet and is extremely resistant to any new foods being added to his diet, consequently his weight is a matter of concern and he also suffers from constipation. Jack's mother, Anne, has to take him to the hospital for regular blood tests to monitor his thyroxine levels and for his weight to be monitored.

Anne worries about trips to the hospital as Jack finds them a source of anxiety. If the trip does not go well, Jack may spend much of the time screaming and running round in circles. This is because the waiting area is often full of people and very noisy and Jack finds crowded places very difficult to be in. Jack is also hypersensitive to noise and the noise level in the waiting room may be causing him some pain, as he covers his ears when he screams.

The behaviour of Jack above may seem extraordinary, yet such apparently extreme responses to hospitalisation in children are not uncommon; nor are the often bemused and helpless reactions of those in the child's vicinity. These individuals, however, are often of course those who are best placed in the situation to help the child avoid such disruptive behaviour and deploy other means of communicating his or her needs. It is hoped here to give the reader not a 'cook-book' of appropriate intervention skills, but to outline a range of useful strategies, which may be adopted by the whole team supplying the child's immediate healthcare needs.

Since the term 'challenging behaviour' is widely used and bears a broad frame of reference, the reader may find it helpful if it is defined before proceeding further. There have, of course, been many attempts to arrive at a definition widely accepted, but that most commonly in use by practitioners in learning disability is that proposed by Emerson:

Culturally abnormal behaviour(s) of such intensity, frequency, or duration that the physical safety of the person or others is likely to be placed in serious jeopardy, or behaviour that is likely to seriously limit use of, or result in the person being denied access to ordinary community facilities.

(Emerson 1995)

The incidence of challenging behaviour in children with disabilities is notably high; Herbert (1993) noted it to be displayed by up to 35 per cent of this population, and to be particularly high in pre-school children experiencing hospitalisation. Other studies have examined the population of children with severe learning disabilities; Chris and Diana Kiernan (1994) identified challenging behaviour in 14 per cent of a large cohort of schoolchildren. Such statistics should not be read as gospel, however, begging as they do questions of definition of the two slippery concepts (challenging behaviour and learning disability) involved; indeed, several authors (Fleming and Kroese 1993; Russell 1997) suggest that whilst the problem is undeniably a common one, reliable statistics are almost impossible to establish. Nevertheless, the conclusion that it is a common phenomenon in hospitalised disabled children is inescapable.

One aspect of these behaviours, however, must be made clear from the start. Bearing in mind the social model of disability outlined in Chapter 2, it is important to stress that the origins of difficult behaviour do not lie solely within the child, but are the product of the child's skills (or lack of them) and the environment – often a *disabling* one – in which he or she is operating. If a non-verbal child wishes to express anxiety in a hospital ward where her customary means of communication are not understood, for example, she may choose aggression as an alternative; behaviour that may result in her being labelled (e.g. as 'violent', or 'aggressive') by uninformed staff, and the subsequent application of punitive, rather than constructive, responses. It is important, therefore, to look for the causes of such behaviours not just within the individual, but also within their environment; these factors have been termed 'settings' by several authors (Zarkowski and Clements 1988; Harris *et al.* 1996).

Developing challenging behaviour

Before examining the potential causes of challenging behaviour in any depth, however, it is important to raise awareness of several general issues. One of these is the factors that result in certain children, regardless of personal or environmental settings, being more 'at risk' of developing challenging behaviours than others. It has been demonstrated, for example, that boys are more likely than girls to communicate externally directed aggression; also that challenging behaviour is more prevalent in children with autism, or sensory impairments (Russell 1997). Children diagnosed with one of a few specific syndromes may also exhibit a raised incidence of problematic behaviour. Examples include Cornelia de Lange syndrome; Prader-Willi syndrome; and Lesch-Nyan syndrome (O'Brien 1998).

Just as there are factors within the child which predispose to challenging behaviour, there are also external factors within the child's experience that may result in a similar bias; indeed the point has been made that it is the interaction between the skills of the child and elements in the environment that produce behaviour of *any* sort (Herbert 1993). The environmental stressors are of course many, but it is possible to review the commonest amongst them here.

Predisposing factors

There are many possible early life events, of course, that predispose to the development of challenging behaviour. These may include: unskilled or insufficient parenting; material or social deprivation; premature separation; and abuse (Russell 1997). Parental death, divorce or separation, whether resulting in single-parent or 'reconstituted' families can also play a part (Herbert 1993), with the child's vulnerability to stress increased by factors including late birth order, family discord, successive health problems, accumulated negative life events and parental low intelligence (ibid.). Families which include a disabled child are, unsurprisingly, more susceptible to internal stress and parental separation (Mencap 1997).

What is most significant to healthcare professionals working with disabled children in hospital, however, is that the experience of hospitalisation, especially if it is repeated, predisposes towards developing difficult behaviour (Herbert 1993). This is particularly so if the child is pre-school, and if the spell in hospital is longer than one week. Sadly, the experience of being in care, albeit less common now for children with disabilities, is also likely to contribute to the development of challenging behaviours (ibid.).

Distressingly for their parents and families, some children diagnosed with particular syndromes demonstrate what are known as 'behavioural phenotypes' (O'Brien 1998). This means that their genetic profile (or genotype) dictates typical patterns of behaviour, which, albeit resistant to intervention, need not be negative; people with Down's syndrome, for example, are characteristically (although not exceptionally) affectionate, fond of music and good mimics. When behavioural phenotypes are generally under discussion, however, it is usually in terms of undesirable traits, often including behaviour that is considered challenging. Children with Lesch-Nyan syndrome, for example, almost invariably present with distressing levels of self-injurious behaviour (O'Brien 1998), and those with Rett's syndrome typically display challenging behaviour related to autistic traits (Mount *et al.* 2001). It is important to stress, however, that whilst the phenotype is 'a characteristic pattern of motor, cognitive, linguistic and social abnormalities . . . consistently associated with a biological disorder' (Flint and Yule 1993), it is *only* 'characteristic'. Not *all* of the behaviours typical of a syndrome will be seen in *all* carriers of the genotype, although all affected individuals will show considerable similarities. Furthermore, although the behaviour may be difficult to treat, there is no reason to suppose that such challenges should be met with a fatalistic or pessimistic response, because observable behaviours are generally the products of interaction between internal and external factors, and where the latter are open to change, all those with ongoing responsibility for the child should be encouraged to seek constructive means of intervention (Berney 1998).

Responding to challenging behaviour

So what, then, is the role of the hospital nurse in responding to the challenging behaviour of a child? It is not likely that staff in the acute care setting will be required to contribute to long-term assessment or planning of interventions, but it is probable that they will be involved in the short-term management of either new or existing behaviours in the child. Many difficult behaviours tend to be situation-specific, or exhibited in response to an unfamiliar environment, such as a hospital (Herbert 1993), and the nurse should be prepared to make all such effort as is necessary first to minimise the risk of such behaviour occurring, and second (if required) to intervene as therapeutically as possible on behalf of the child. It may be recalled that collaborative working, especially with families, is central to the stipulations of the Children Act (ibid.), and before any action is taken in the hospital setting it is discussed with the child's carers as a matter of priority. Indeed, any interventions already in place are likely to have been founded on the principle that sees the parents as therapists (Russell 1997). The discussion with the family (or other prime carers) should embrace all the key elements of the assessment and intervention structure set out below.

There is no space here to discuss either the principles or detail of various behavioural approaches (for both, see Russell 1997; Zarkowski and Clements 1988), but it is hoped to give the reader sufficient information to allow him or her to work with others in responding to the behaviour in a knowledgeable and confident manner that takes due account of United Kingdom law (the Children Act discussed here only pertains in England and Wales, but Scotland and Northern Ireland have made very similar provision).

The Children Act

It would be useful therefore at this point to examine the parameters laid down by the Children Act in working with children in this context. It may come as a surprise to learn that the Act makes no specific mention of disabled children with challenging behaviour (Russell 1997), but there are provisions for children 'in need', the further description of whom clearly includes the former group. The final responsibility for services for this group lies with local authorities, also bound to work in partnership with families and other significant agencies; the hospital nurse is affected only by the need for awareness of how any long-term behaviour of the child should be addressed elsewhere, and an awareness of the legality of any physical interventions adopted in the acute setting.

Local authorities are required under the Act to identify children in need within their area, make due service provision for them, work collaboratively with families and other relevant agencies and take steps to protect children identified as being at risk. The Act also seeks to achieve a balance in law between the child's welfare and the rights and responsibilities of the parents (Herbert 1993). Little of this may appear relevant to the nurse confronted by an intensely uncooperative child resisting some intervention vital to his or her well-being, yet it is essential to remember that it is the Children Act that provides the framework by which all agencies should work to meet the needs of that child.

Restraint

The contents of the Act become more directly relevant when it comes to issues of control and restraint. Two of the main emphases lie on the rights and responsibilities of parents, and on the ultimate welfare of the child, stipulating that any intervention adopted by parents or professionals should always be in the latter's 'paramount interests' (Russell 1997). It goes without saying that children with multiple disabilities are amongst the most vulnerable in our society, and that therefore protection from abuse should be every involved professional's highest priority. Many of the physical interventions demanded in the acute setting may either in themselves bring risk of abuse, or the constraints needed to perform them may do so. Despite the best intentions of the Children Act, it has been reported that its provisions in this context at times are unclear and give rise to varieties of interpretation (Russell 1997) in practice.

In response, the Mental Health Foundation has issued guidelines for professionals (Lyon 1994a) and carers (Lyon 1994b), which aim to clarify several areas of confusion. It must be stated, however, that amongst the invaluable practical advice in the documents, there is also Professor Lyon's admission that the legality of some very specific interventions would have to be tested in the courts.

Both sets of guidelines set out three main principles which should guide the use of control and restraint – measures which otherwise carry risk of abuse, and which have been considerably misused with people with learning disabilities in the past (Ryan and Thomas 1993). These principles are:

- Physical interventions should only be used as a last resort to respond to challenging behaviour, and only in the least harmful manner and for the shortest possible time. Never should they be used as a result of pressures upon time or staffing.

- Any physical interventions adopted should form part of an existing care plan that has been discussed with parents by all other agencies concerned.
- Interventions should be regularly reviewed to evaluate their effectiveness for the individual (Russell 1997).

This guidance is echoed by the National Autistic Society and the British Institute of Learning Disabilities in their authoritative work on physical interventions, which although designed to meet the needs of adults, is nevertheless applicable to children in the institutional setting (Harris *et al*. 1996), and which the reader may find particularly helpful in its detail on key principles.

More directly relevant guidance is that produced by the Royal College of Nursing (1999), which distinguishes between restraint (action taken to overpower the child, necessarily without consent), holding still (immobilisation, which uses less force and may be deployed with the child's permission) and containment (means to prevent the child leaving, or seriously damaging themselves or property). The document repeats the broad principles of both the Children Act and the Mental Health Foundation, but in addition states that any action taken should be based on a policy relevant to the particular client group and setting, and that sufficient numbers of staff should be adequately trained in the necessary techniques. It also states that services should make allowance for those members of staff who may dissent from specific action agreed – an important provision in an area that can sometimes seem an ethical minefield. The detail of the RCN's recommendations is invaluable, and the reader is strongly urged to consult the document for themselves.

Preventing and managing challenging behaviour

It is perhaps an obvious point that the best way to manage challenging behaviour in children (or adults) is to prevent it happening in the first place; but it is nevertheless worth spending some time in consideration of the potentially most valuable strategies to this end. In the long term, truly effective prevention requires assessment of the individual to the extent that at least a certain amount of the behaviour becomes predictable (Emerson 1995). In the context of the acute setting it is unlikely that this will be possible, and the nursing staff will be thrown somewhat onto their own resources (and that of the family) in order to be able to tackle the problem. Since much challenging behaviour is context-specific, it follows that manipulation of the factors which contribute to maintaining the behaviour will have some effect (hopefully positive!) on the likelihood of that behaviour recurring (ibid.).

Emerson (1995) has suggested that there are three broad aspects to developing prevention strategies, each of which should have been exposed in a 'functional' assessment of the individual (i.e. an assessment that clarifies the function that the behaviour serves for the subject – such as the accumulation of evidence to show that a child habitually pinches people in order to maintain her personal space). These three areas involve identification of:

- The 'settings' (or situations) in which the behaviour is most likely to occur.
- The personal or environmental events which operate within the above to instigate or prevent the behaviour occurring.
- The nature of the contingencies maintaining the behaviour.

The accurate isolation of the factors involving the three areas above can then be used to 're-schedule' the individual's activities (to avoid the conditions in which the behaviour is most likely to occur), and/or to 'modify' setting events (Emerson 1995). The first case is difficult to implement, of course, in the acute setting; but an example might be the provision of the child's favourite music in a private room where he has begun to self-injure as a result of anxiety in the unfamiliar surroundings. An example of the second would be to desensitise the child to stressful procedures (e.g. routine injections) by means of pictures, discussion, demonstration or whatever other methods necessary before the real event occurs.

Even with the deployment of the most sensitive prevention strategies, however, it is not unlikely that multiply disabled children will still exhibit problematic behaviour in the acute care setting, and it would be timely now to consider the most appropriate responses. In doing so, the reader is reminded that the intention here is not to cover the proposed ground in as much detail as they may feel the practice situation requires (for that they are referred to the authorities given), but only to give an outline of how responses might be governed.

Intervention options

There are of course many different ways in which behaviour considered challenging may be approached. These may include straightforward 'behavioural' methods (where the principles of operant learning, or cause and effect, are deployed), pharmacological interventions (usually urged as a last resort, or in combination with other methods, Clarke 1993) or alternative means, such as 'gentle teaching' (Harbridge 1992) or aromatherapy. In practice, it is common for professionals to combine two or more techniques, but the fundamental principles of intervention invariably apply.

It will be recalled that interventions used in the past to modify the difficult behaviour of individuals with learning disabilities were often at best morally suspect, and at worst downright abusive (Ryan and Thomas 1993); but although the extremes of behaviour modification are now largely history, techniques based on the approach (as well as other potentially abusive methods) are still very much in use and thus in need of a stringent ethical framework if they are to be utilised in the best interests of the client. It is to this end that Emerson (1995) set out his tripartite structure for the bases of intervention, one of which every healthcare professional aiming to meet the needs of challenging individuals should be aware of. The proposal was that therapeutic approaches to the management of challenging behaviour should be founded upon three principles.

The first of these is that the approach should be *constructional*. By this is meant that the primary goal should not be to eradicate a behaviour, so much as to construct a repertoire of more acceptable responses to the same 'settings'. For example, it might be considered valid to teach the pinching child mentioned above other non-verbal means of signifying her dislike of the proximity of others, such as holding out her hand in a gesture of rebuttal.

The second principle put forward by Emerson is that of the necessary *functional* basis of any planned intervention. This demands that any approach to the individual's behaviour be based upon an assessment that has accurately established the precipitating and maintaining factors behind it. Few healthcare professionals prescribe medication for symptoms without first making a diagnosis, and this principle is an exact parallel. Only when the function that the child's habitual pinching serves for her has been identified can a realistic approach to replacing the aggression with more appropriate behaviour be adopted.

Finally, Emerson proposes that any intervention planned should be *socially valid*. This indicates that the method adopted should (a) tackle behaviour that is socially significant in its undesirability, (b) involve means, which are acceptable to all parties involved and (c) produce socially desirable consequences. Only if such an approach is followed can the abuses of the past, which involved not only the harshest methods, but also the 'treatment' of some fairly insignificant behaviours, be avoided.

It should be remembered that any long-term behaviour of the child that is considered challenging should already be addressed, prior to hospital admission, by a plan of intervention drawn up in collaboration between parents and professionals; in the acute setting, this should either be followed in the exact manner as it is elsewhere, or, if really necessary, adapted to the novelty of the child's temporary surroundings. Any adaptation should be effected by ward staff in consultation with all those involved in the original assessment and plan.

Some behaviours witnessed by nursing staff, however, are likely to be 'new' to the child, or at least appear (on assessment and in consultation with the parents) to be specific to the hospital context. In this case, it will be necessary to assess the behaviours as speedily as possible, but maintaining accuracy as a priority using the functional approach outlined by Emerson. When this has been done, a plan for intervention can be established with the aid of the child's principal carers, one that initially seeks to prevent the behaviour occurring in the first place. Should methods of prevention fail or prove unrealistic in the hospital setting, then a collaborative decision will need to be made about the need to intervene in a therapeutic manner. It could be, for instance, that the assessment has shown that the behaviour is so very specific to the context, that the short time that the child is expected to be hospitalised does not warrant any further intervention.

Should it be established that a planned therapeutic response will be in the best interests of the child, nursing staff should be at the forefront of the team approach. It should not be envisaged that these individuals will be best equipped to generate a skilled response based upon relevant knowledge, skills and experience; this rather should be the preserve of the community learning disability team, preferably in the person of its member who already provides a service to the child (probably a learning disability nurse).

Referrals may generally be made on an informal basis to the local team, and need not be diverted through any other health professional. Unless the behaviour of the child presents as a serious crisis, however, it is unlikely that any member of the team will be able to respond in person to the referral as soon as those supporting the child would like. In that case, it will be necessary to seek a telephone consultation only, and hospital staff would do best to take the advice of the child's community keyworker, or at least that of a learning disability professional, working in collaboration with the family in order to develop the most appropriate response to the behaviour.

As indicated, it has not been possible here to give the reader a comprehensive guide to interventions based on behavioural, pharmacological or alternative means. For these, they are referred to Emerson (1995), Clarke (1993) and Harbridge (1992) respectively. It is hoped, however, that this chapter has given sufficient insight into the most appropriate and productive frameworks for intervening therapeutically to reduce the distress for the child of behaviours such as Jack's above.

References

Berney, T. P. (1998) ' "Born to . . ." – Genetics and Behaviour' *British Journal of Learning Disabilities*, 26(1) 4–8.

Clarke, D. (1993) 'Psychopharmacological approaches to challenging behaviour' in I. Fleming and B. S. Kroese (eds) *People with learning disability and severe challenging behaviour*, Manchester: Manchester University Press.

Emerson, E. (1995) *Challenging Behaviour: Analysis and Intervention in People with Learning Difficulties*, Cambridge: Cambridge University Press.

Fleming, I. and Kroese, B. S. (eds) (1993) *People with learning disability and severe challenging behaviour: New developments in services and therapy*, Manchester: Manchester University Press.

Flint, J. and Yule, W. (1993) 'Behavioural Phenotypes', in M. Rutter and L. Hersov (eds), *Recent Advances in Child and Adolescent Psychiatry*, (3rd edn) Oxford: Blackwell Scientific.

Harbridge, E. (1992) *Learning Together; How Gentle Teaching helps people with challenging behaviour*, Minehead: Hexagon.

Harris, J., Allen, D., Cornick, M., Jefferson, A. and Mills, R. (1996) *Physical Interven-*

tions: A Policy Framework, Kidderminster: British Institute of Learning Disability and National Autistic Society.

Herbert, M. (1993) *Working with Children and the Children Act*, Leicester: British Psychological Society.

Kiernan, C. and Kiernan, D. (1994) 'Challenging behaviour in schools for pupils with severe learning disabilities' *Mental Handicap Research* 7, 117–201.

Lyon, C. (1994a) *Legal issues arising from the care, control and safety of children with learning disabilities who also present severe challenging behaviour: Policy and Guidance*, London: Mental Health Foundation.

Lyon, C. (1994b) *Legal issues arising from the care, control and safety of children with learning disabilities who also present severe challenging behaviour: A Guide for Parents and Carers*, London: Mental Health Foundation.

Mencap (1997) *Left in the Dark: a Mencap report on the challenges facing the UK's 400,000 families of children with learning disabilities*, London: Mencap.

Mount, R. H., Hastings, R. P., Reilly, S., Cass, H. and Charman, T. (2001) 'Behavioural and emotional features in Rett syndrome', *Disability and Rehabilitation* 23(3/4) 129–138.

O'Brien, G. (1998) 'Behavioural Phenotypes', in M. Kerr (ed.) *Innovations in Health Care for People with Intellectual Disabilities*, Chorley: Lisieux Hall.

Royal College of Nursing (1999) *Restraining, Holding Still and Containing Children*, London: RCN.

Ryan, J. and Thomas, F. (1993) Chapter 3 in *The Politics of Mental Handicap*, London: Free Association Books.

Russell, P. (ed.) (1997) *Don't Forget Us: Children with Learning Disabilities and Severe Challenging Behaviour*: London: Mental Health Foundation.

Zarkowski, E. and Clements, J. (1988) *Problem behaviour in people with severe learning disabilities: A practical guide to a constructional approach*, Beckenham: Croom Helm.

13 The importance of appropriate respite care

Claire Thurgate

Still, children with disabilities are being inappropriately admitted to acute wards, or having their admissions prolonged so that their families can receive a break from caring. What these families need, rather than blocking beds on already busy wards, is appropriate respite that gives them a chance to find the energy within themselves, and support in others to devote attention to their children. This chapter will aim to discuss the impact on families of caring for a child with disabilities; the process model of stress and caring; how the concept of respite arose and what is respite; settings in which respite is provided; characteristics of families and children accessing respite; the advantages and disadvantages of respite for families and children and accessing respite.

Impact on families of caring for a child with a disability

The stereotyped notion of 'the family' with two married parents of the opposite sex, two children, and the father as the sole wage earner is a reality for fewer and fewer (Carpenter 1998; Dale 1996). Knox *et al.* (2000) believe that the family is a 'complex and dynamic system with its own characteristics and needs . . . comprised of individual members who also have their own unique characters and needs'. Perhaps this is a more appropriate concept where the 'forms' rather than the 'functions' of the family are changing (Dahlstrom 1989, cited in Carpenter 1998). Dale (1996) has identified three models for understanding the family – The pathological model, The Common Needs model and The Stress/Coping model which are presented in Table 13.1.

Impact of caring on mothers In most families it is the mother who will become the main carer (Carpenter 1998; Bowyer and Hayes 1998; Read 2000). Quine and Pahl (1991) believe that mothers become stressed at being at home giving constant care, with the home being likened to a prison (Brinchmann 1999). However, Bowyer and Hayes (1998) in a study on mothering in families with and without a child with disabilities found that feelings of vulnerability are not exclusive to mothers whose child has a disability.

Table 13.1 Framework for understanding the family

Model	Definition

The Pathological Model	Any difficulties in a family member stem from having a child with special needs in the family.
	    The birth of a disabled child was seen as a 'crisis', and this concept of 'crisis' was extended to the family.
	    This model has been important for thinking about some of the adverse effects of a child with special needs on the family.

The Common Needs Model	Instead of seeing the child as pathology, unmet needs for services and material resources (*deficits*) were a major source of stress.
The Stress/Coping Model	Main finding is the *variability* in coping within and between individuals over time. Many families cope remarkably well and show no apparent differences from ordinary families in the community (Byrne *et al.* 1988, cited in Dale 1996).

Source: adapted from Dale (1996).

Impact of caring on fathers The birth of a child with disability will also bring life-transforming experiences for fathers (Meyer 1995, cited in Carpenter 1998). Some fathers may display aspects of their personality that had not previously been acknowledged, while others experience 'relentless stress'. Interestingly, in a New Zealand study by Bray (1995, cited by Carpenter 1998) the cohort of fathers displayed two types of love. There were those who displayed utter devotion, whilst others felt they could perform transforming acts, and transform their child. However, when it came to caring for their child with disabilities, Atkin (1992, cited in Read 2000) found that fathers performed some of the practical and physical jobs, but this did not include personal care. This may have further implications on the mothers' caring role.

Impact of caring on siblings It is generally agreed, within the literature, that having a child with disabilities can have a detrimental effect on siblings. The sibling may display behavioural changes, increased responsibility and feelings of neglect (Klein-Berndt 1991 and Procter *et al.* 1998 cited in Murphy 2001). On the other hand, Byrne *et al.* 1988 (cited in Carpenter 1998) found that siblings showed no difference in emotional and behavioural disturbances to siblings of 'normal' children. This is supported by Dale (1996), who also found that siblings were well adjusted, and mature and showed a responsible attitude, which went beyond their chronological age, though it must be asked if this could be detrimental to the child.

Social, financial and emotional cost of caring As well as impacting on individual family members, caring for a child with disabilities also places social, financial and emotional costs on the family. Throughout the literature, social isolation is a constant theme (Jennings 1990; Teague *et al.* 1993; Patterson *et al.* 1994). This isolation may be the result of medicalisation of the home, which subsequently threatens the family's intimacy, security and comfort of home life, while the constant input of professionals may contribute to a lack of privacy for the family (Patterson *et al.* 1994). This situation could be exacerbated due to lack of babysitters thus restricting the family's activities outside of the home. A lack of freedom may have a financial impact on the family, as one parent, usually the mother, will give up a job to care for the child with a disability. Added financial costs, over and above caring for a non-disabled child, may be felt by the family including aids to adapt the house, increased laundry and extra equipment. Consequently, the impact of having a child with a disability, together with the social and financial implications may increase the emotional burden on the family. This view is supported by Kirk (1998), who feels that the emotional cost of caring is a constant theme in the literature and may be depicted as sleep deprivation, stress and depression. Therefore, it is important to understand how individuals may adjust to meet these stressors. The process model of stress and coping (Lazarus and Folkman 1984, cited in Beresford and Sloper 1999) is a widely accepted and valid way of understanding the relationship between individual's adjustment.

The process model of stress and coping

The process model of stress and coping has two basic components to the coping process – appraisal and the use of coping strategies. These aspects are subsequently influenced by factors which are known collectively as coping resources. Burr and Klein (1994, cited in Taanila *et al.* 2002) have developed a conceptual framework of coping strategies (See Table 13.2).

One outcome of the coping process is adaptation (Lazarus and Folkman 1984, cited in Beresford and Sloper 1999) which is defined as the degree to which parents cope psychologically, socially and physically with the health needs of their child (Hentinen and Kyngas 1998). Interestingly, Hentinen and Kyngas (1998) in their study of 189 families found that good adaptation includes acceptance of the situation, good relationships between family members, freedom to express feelings in the family and few or no problems in taking care of the child. On the other hand, poor adaptation included conflict within the family, their attitude to their child with disability differed from the attitude to the healthy siblings and the family had problems in caring for the child. Parents who presented with poor adaptation believed that they received poor emotional and instrumental support from relatives and poor support from health professionals (Hentinen and Kyngas 1998). For families to care for their child with disabilities at home it is important that appropriate support services are provided. The provision of respite is one such service.

Table 13.2 The conceptual framework of coping strategies

Highly abstract strategies	Moderately abstract strategies
Cognitive	Be accepting of the situation and others Gain useful knowledge Change how the situation is viewed or defined (reframe the situation)
Emotional	Express feelings and affection Be sensitive to others' emotional needs Avoid or resolve negative feelings and disabling expressions of emotions
Relationships	Increase cohesion Increase adaptability Develop increased trust Increase cooperation Increase tolerance of each other
Communication	Be open and honest Listen to each other Be sensitive to non-verbal communication
Community	Seek help and support from others Fulfil expectations in organisations
Spiritual	Be more involved in religious activities Increase faith or seek help from God
Individual development	Develop autonomy, independence and self-sufficiency Keep active in hobbies

Source: adapted from Burr and Klein (1994).

Respite

The impact of the NHS and Community Care Act (1990) was that children with disabilities, who had hitherto been cared for in institutions, would now be able to live 'ordinary lives' within the community with services tailored to meet their individual needs. This view is reinforced by the Children Act (1989) which highlights the need for children to live within a family environment as the family has a unique knowledge and understanding of the child's individual needs. It is also felt that the family home is the most natural place for a child to grow and develop. While advocating for the child with disabilities to be cared for within the community, the NHS and Community Care Act (1990) and the Children Act (1989) highlight the need for families to be supported.

Unfortunately, for many children and their families support was initially achieved through inappropriate admissions to children's wards (Oswin 1985, cited in Baldwin and Carlisle 1994; Campbell 1996; Olsen and Maslin-Prothero 2001) which, understandably, parents were dissatisfied with. Consequently, two alternative forms of support were identified – the provision of short-term care in residential units which is preferred by some families as it is always there and is felt to be reliable (Morris 1998) and the development of family-based care which may offer families more flexibility (ibid. 1998).

There are numerous definitions of the term 'respite' with Treneman *et al.* (1997) believing that respite involves the shared care of a person with difficulties either at home or in a residential setting in order to give the family a break from caring. Treneman *et al.* (1997) respect that families need to have a break from caring as the burden of caring with ineffective support affects parental well-being and ultimately family wellness (Beresford 1994; Prilleltensky and Nelson 2000). However, they omit to mention whether respite benefits the child, and that the child is a burden to the family, a point reinforced by Middleton (1999) who suggests that the term 'respite' supports the idea that the child is a problem for the family rather than an individual with its own needs. Laverty and Reet's (2001) definition may be more appropriate as they believe that respite should provide therapeutic opportunity, quality time, independence and the living of life for all family members – 'a gift of time for both the child and their family' (ibid.). This definition embraces the child and its family as a whole and encompasses the need for respite to provide the child with opportunities, rather than just providing the family with a break from caring. In order to achieve this respite needs to be more flexible and to respond to individual families' needs (Murray 2000; Miller 2002; Department of Health 1996,1998).

Characteristic of families and children accessing respite

It appears from the research that the majority of parents accessing respite are over forty years of age (Hoare *et al.* 1998; Neufeld, Query and Drummond 2001; McConkey and Adams 2000). It is difficult to understand why mainly parents over forty access respite. It may be that they are better able to demand it, they have more demands on them so need respite or because of older maternal age have more high-risk pregnancies. It also appears that parents accessing respite are likely to be married (Hoare *et al.* 1998; McConkey and Adams 2000; While *et al.* 1996 and Taanila *et al.* 2002), though it is difficult to determine if respite has a role in preventing marital breakdown. However, caring for a child with disabilities may affect the family's financial situation. This may be in part due to the extra costs of having a child with disabilities as well as the impact on earnings as no more than 50 per cent of mothers, whose child was accessing respite, were in employment (Cowen and Reed 2002). Unfortunately, Cowen and Reed (2002) fail to discuss whether the mothers would have worked had their child not had a disability, or whether these figures were common to all mothers. Consequently, it is important for respite services to have an understanding of the financial pressures faced by families so that appropriate information regarding support may be given. For some parents the stress of caring for a child with disabilities may affect their mental health (Hoare *et al.* 1998; Sherman 1995). However, it must be noted in Sherman's (1995) study that the mean age of the child was three, and stress could be attributed to having a pre-school child at home. It appears that the child's characteristics such as physical dependence, locomotor disability, mobility, toileting dependency, sleep dif- ficulties, behavioural problems and communication were the main stressors for some families (Hoare *et al.* 1998; Treneman *et al.* 1997).

Children accessing respite care present with a number of different charac- teristics. Interestingly, Hoare *et al.* (1998) found that the majority of chil- dren presented with challenging behaviours – poor sleep (59 per cent), screaming (32 per cent) and aggression towards themselves and others (32 per cent). On the other hand, the results of Neufeld *et al.* (2001) showed that children in respite required assistance with everyday activities (59 per cent), needed regular medication (41 per cent) and technology to maintain everyday functions (35 per cent). These findings support Treneman *et al.* (1997) who found a significant relationship between the amount of help that the child required with everyday activities and the amount of respite accessed. Consequently, it may be more appropriate to provide effective support within the child's home, to aid activities, rather than place the child in overnight respite.

Advantages and disadvantages of respite

Stalker and Robinson (1994) found that the principle effects of respite, iden- tified by parents, were the opportunity to relax and a decreased feeling of stress (43%–48%). Interestingly, there was no difference between the extent and nature of benefits and the service accessed. However, Stalker and Robin- son (1994) included a table (See Table 13.3) in their study highlighting the benefits of respite for the family. This shows that for the majority of families Health Authority respite allows for more social or work activities than either family or local authority schemes. It also highlights that local authority res- pite had the least effect for families – 6.1 per cent compared to 2.0 per cent for health authority respite. It is difficult to understand why this may be, as no qualitative data is included in the study.

Interestingly, McConkey and Adams (2000) showed different results to Stalker and Robinson (1994) with family breaks benefiting 86 per cent of families while hospital breaks benefited only 47 per cent. The difference between the two studies may be attributed to the fact that Stalker and Robin- son's data was collected from parents whilst the data in McConkey and Adams (2000) was collected by social workers who may have had different perceptions from parents. Meanwhile, Olsen and Maslin-Prothero (2001), studying the effect of in-home respite found that of 17 families only 5 attrib- uted improvements in family wellness to respite. These findings, and to a lesser extent the findings of Stalker and Robinson (1994) and McConkey and Adams (2000), suggest that respite support is important for some families,

Table 13.3 Reported benefits to the family

Benefits	Family-based scheme % of responses	Local Authority residential % of responses	Health Authority % of responses
Relaxation/less stress	43.8	48.5	43.1
Improved family relations	30.5	26.3	27.5
Allows for social or work activities	19	17.2	25.5
Helps the child only	1.9	–	2.0
Negative effect only	1.9	2.0	–
No effect	2.9	6.1	2.0
Totals	100	100	100

Source: Stalker and Robinson (1994).

but for many it is maybe only one of a variety of factors in determining improvements in family wellness. This endorses other research, which has questioned the extent to which respite contributes to the longer well-being of carers (McNally *et al.* 1999).

It is acknowledged in the research that respite gives parents a break from caring (McGill 1996), but what is difficult to ascertain is what length of respite is considered to be adequate. Neufeld *et al.* (2001) in their research found that there was no association between amount of respite and the perception of an adequate break. However, Sherman (1995) found that higher rates of utilisation were significantly associated with lower sibling strain and lower expressed somatisation. The above findings reiterate that each family is individual with differing circumstances, which need to be acknowledged when planning and executing respite. It also highlights the need for further research to be undertaken in how respite is allocated.

Not only does respite have advantages and disadvantages for families, but also the children who access it. Minkes *et al.* (1994) found that children undertook a range of activities and the majority enjoyed their stay. The findings from Stalker and Robinson's (1994) study are presented in Table 13.4. Interestingly, only 7 per cent of families accessing health authority facilities perceive more freedom/independence for their child compared to 25 per cent and 22.8 per cent respectively for family and local authority provisions. Health authority provisions also had no benefits for 27.9 per cent of families compared to 1.8 per cent and 7.9 per cent respectively for family-based and local authority provisions.

Minkes *et al.* (1994) identified problems with respite which included a lack of choice, especially when choosing food and little contact with non-disabled children. This will not only affect the child's independence skills, but also prevents social inclusion.

Table 13.4 Perceived benefit to the child of using different respite services

Type of benefit	Family-based scheme % of responses	Local Authority residential % of responses	Health Authority % of responses
More freedom/independence	25.0	22.8	7.0
Chance to mix with other adults	23.2	19.8	16.3
Chance to mix with other children	12.5	15.8	13.9
Outings	8.9	2.0	–
New skills	5.4	6.9	2.3
Chance to develop close relationships	4.5	3.0	2.3
Improved behaviour	1.8	5.0	4.7
Pleasure/attention	4.5	4.0	2.3
New experiences	7.1	7.9	11.6
Better health	0.9	1.0	–
Returns to better environment	4.5	3.0	7.0
Too soon to say	–	1.0	4.7
None	1.8	7.9	27.9
Totals	100	100	100

Source: Stalker and Robinson (1994).

Accessing respite

Five themes, pertaining to accessing respite, emerge from the literature – choice/suitability, utilisation, more care, communication and staff.

The first theme, choice/suitability found that appropriate respite facilities are dependent upon the characteristics of the child and the family (McConkey and Adams 2000). Residential units were 'extremely valuable' for children who were not aware of dangers (62 per cent compared to 33 per cent of those who were aware) and for those who were highly dependent (67 per cent compared to 20 per cent of low dependent children). Breakaways were valuable for 75 per cent of families with children under 10 compared to 47 per cent of families with children aged 11–16. Hospitals, meanwhile, were valuable if children weren't aware of common dangers (27 per cent v 3 per cent) and had behaviour problems (28 per cent v 7 per cent). Although McConkey and Adams (2000) study highlights the need for suitable respite provision, it fails to address whether, from a parental perspective, the respite service meets the child's needs, and the importance of suitable respite provision. Despite these findings, many families have difficulty in accessing suitable respite services, while a number of families access more than one service (Robinson *et al*. 2001).

In two studies Robinson *et al*. (2001) found that between 18 per cent and 28 per cent of children access two or more forms of residential respite. Interestingly, these findings are similar to those of McConkey and Adams

(2000) who found that 17 per cent of children access two or more facilities for overnight care. Unfortunately, it is not known what effect, either positive or negative, this may have on the child. Therefore, it may be appropriate to undertake a study to ascertain the effects, for the child, of accessing multi-respite services. The question that must be asked if some children access more than one respite service is do they receive more respite than those that only access one service?

When it comes to enough care, Treneman *et al.* (1997) found that only 17 per cent of families received almost enough respite, 35 per cent were satisfied with the amount they received while 50 per cent wanted more. However, from a social worker's perspective (McConkey and Adams 2000) 69 per cent of families were in need of more care, while only 11 per cent of families instanced 'more respite' highlighting the difference between professionals and parental perceptions. It is also difficult to ascertain what is meant by 'enough' respite as each family has its own unique needs and perception of these needs. As well as highlighting the need for more care families want more appropriate information from respite services.

Unfortunately, a lack of information was the most frequent reason for dissatisfaction with respite (Treneman *et al.* 1997). Parents also want better information and feedback following respite (Stalker and Robinson 1994). These findings are supported by Brodin and Paulin (1997), who found that many families lacked information. Other issues regarding information include wanting to have a say and to be listened to (McGill 1996) and to be better informed about available respite options (Robinson *et al.* 2001; Campbell 1996). Although these three studies have small samples they highlight the problems in communication in respite settings throughout the UK. Poor communication with professionals was also perceived as a stressor for parents. Consequently, closer liaison is required between health, social services and education (Campbell 1996), which may be achieved through joint working. Respite services must also ensure that appropriately qualified staff (Neufeld *et al.* 2001; Robinson *et al.* 2001; McGill 1996; Petr *et al.* 1995; Brodin and Paulin 1997) care for the children that the families are able to trust (Valkenier *et al.* 2002; Stalker and Robinson 1994).

Recommendations for practice

- Families require suitable respite, which is available and flexible to meet the child's and their individual needs. Short notice and emergency care must also be available to support families at times of 'crisis'.
- It is imperative that equality of respite services is available to all families, and not just those who shout the loudest. This may be achieved through multi-agency panels, which are able to monitor respite usage, and act as a gate keeper.
- Providers of respite services need to be innovative, so that the service

responds to the child and family's needs, and not the child and family to the service need. For example, it may be more appropriate to provide a carer to go on holiday with the family, rather than the child being separated from the family in residential care.

- For many families accessing respite can be a stressful experience, so it is essential to ensure that the child and their family are appropriately prepared for their first visit. This should be an individual programme based on each family's needs, making it family led and not service led.
- An important component of respite care is effective and appropriate communication. This must not only involve the family but also the multi-disciplinary team involved with the child's care, thus ensuring that the child receives individualised and appropriate care and any issues or concerns can be dealt with at an early stage. Effective communication may be achieved through verbal handovers after the child's stay which are reinforced through the use of communication books; communication passports; annual respite reviews; liaison with the multi-disciplinary team which should also include social services and education; quarterly newsletters; family get-togethers, and events for siblings.
- It is important that respite is not a service in isolation, but is an integral part of the team around the child with disabilities.

References

Baldwin, S. and Carlisle, J. (1994) 'Social support for disabled children and their families: A review of the literature', Social Work Services Inspectorate, Edinburgh: HMSO.

Beresford, B. (1994) *Positively parents: caring for a severely disabled child*, York: Social Policy Research Unit, University of York.

Beresford, B. and Sloper, T. (1999) *The information needs of chronically ill or physically disabled children and adolescents*, York: Social Policy Research Unit.

Bowyer, A. and Hayes, A. (1998) 'Mothering in families with and without a child with disability', *International Journal of Disability, Development and Education*, 45(3) 313–322.

Brinchmann, B. (1999) 'When the home becomes a prison: living with a severely disabled child', *Nursing Ethics*, 6(2) 137–143.

Brodin, J. and Paulin, S. (1997) 'Parents' views of respite care services for families with children with disabilities in Sweden', *European Journal of Special Needs Education*, 12(3) 197–205.

Campbell, H. (1996) 'Inter-agency assessment of respite care needs of families of children with special needs in Fife', *Public Health*, 110, 151–155.

Carpenter, B. (1998) 'Defining the family: towards a critical framework for families of children with disabilities', *European Journal of Special Needs Education*, 13(2) 180–188.

Cowen, P. and Reed, D. (2002) 'Effects of respite care for children with developmental disabilities: an evaluation of an intervention for at risk families', *Public Health Nursing*, 19(4) 272–283.

Dale, N. (1996) *Working with families of children with special needs – partnership and practice*, London: Routledge.

Department of Health (1989) *The Children Act*, London: HMSO.

Department of Health (1990) *The National Health Service and Community Care Act*, London: HMSO.

Department of Health (1996) *Child health in the community: a guide to good practice*, London: HMSO.

Department of Health (1998) *Evaluation of the pilot project programme for children with life threatening illnesses*, London: NHS Executive.

Hentinen, M. and Kyngas, H. (1998) 'Factors associated with the adaptation of parents with a chronically ill child', *Journal of Clinical Nursing*, 7, 316–324.

Hoare, P., Harris, M., Jackson, P. and Kerley, S. (1998) 'A community survey of children with severe intellectual disability and their families: psychological adjustment, carer distress and the effect of respite care', *Journal of Intellectual Disability Research*, 42(3) 218–227.

Jennings, P. (1990) 'Caring for a child with a tracheotomy', *Nursing Standard*, 4(30) 24–26 and 4(32) 38–40.

Kirk, S. (1998) 'Families' experiences of caring at home for a technology-dependent child: a review of the literature', *Child: Care, Health and Development*, 24(2) 101–114.

Knox, M., Parmenter, T., Atkinson, N. and Yazbeck, M. (2000) 'Family control: the views of families who have a child with an intellectual disability', *Journal of Applied Research in Intellectual Disabilities*, 13, 1–16.

Laverty, H. and Reet, M. (2001) *Planning care for children in respite settings*, London: Jessica Kingsley.

McConkey, R. and Adams, L. (2000) 'Matching short break services for children with learning disabilities to family needs and preferences', *Child: Care, Health and Development*, 26(5) 429–444.

McGill, P. (1996) 'Summer holiday respite provision for the families of children and young people with learning disabilities', *Child: Care, Health and Development*, 22(3) 203–212.

McNally, S., Ben-Sholom, Y. and Newman, S. (1999) 'The effects of respite care on informal carers' well-being: a systematic review', *Disability and Rehabilitation*, 21, 1–14.

Middleton, L. (1999) *Disabled children: Challenging social exclusion*, London: Blackwell Science.

Miller, S. (2002) 'Respite care for children who have complex health needs', *Paediatric Nursing*, 14(5) 33–37.

Minkes, J., Robinson, C. and Weston, C. (1994) 'Consulting the children: interviews with children using residential respite care services', *Disability and Society*, 9(1) 47–57.

Morris, J. (1998) *Still Missing. Vol. 2: disabled children and The Children Act*, London: The Who Cares? Trust.

Murphy, G. (2001) 'The technology–dependent child at home: Part 1: In whose best interest?', *Paediatric Nursing*, 13(7) 14–18.

Murray, P. (2000) 'Disabled children, parents and professionals: Partnership on whose terms?' *Disability and Society* 15(4) 683–698.

Neufeld S., Query, B. and Drummond, J. (2001) 'Respite care users who have children with chronic conditions: are they getting a break?' *Journal of Pediatric Nursing*, 16 (4) 234–243.

Olsen, R. and Maslin-Prothero, P. (2001) 'Dilemmas in the provision of own home respite support for parents of young children with complex healthcare needs: evidence from an evaluation', *Journal of Advanced Nursing*, 34(5) 603–610.

Patterson, J., Jernell, J., Leonard, B. and Titus, J. (1994) 'Caring for medically fragile children at home: the parent professional relationship', *Journal of Pediatric Nursing*, 9(2) 98–106.

Petr, C. *et al.* (1995) 'Home Care for children dependent on medical technology: The family perspective', *Social Work in Healthcare* 21(1) 5–22.

Prilleltensky, I. and Nelson, G. (2000) 'Promoting child and family wellness: priorities for psychological and social interventions', *Journal of Community and Applied Social Psychology*, 10, 85–105.

Quine, L. and Pahl, J. (1991) 'Stress and coping in mothers caring for a child with severe learning difficulties: a Test of Lazarus' Transaction model of coping', *Journal of Community and Applied Social Psychology*, 1(1) 57–70.

Read, J. (2000) *Disability, the family and society*, Buckingham: Open University Press.

Robinson, C., Jackson, P. and Townsley, R. (2001) 'Short breaks for families caring for a disabled child with complex health needs', *Child and Family Social Work*, 6, 67–75.

Sherman, B. (1995) 'Impact of home-based respite care on families of children with chronic illnesses', *Children's Health Care*, 24(1) 33–45.

Sloper, P. and Turner, S. (1992) 'Service needs of families and children with severe physical disability, *Child: Care, Health and Development*, 18, 259–282.

Stalker, K. and Robinson, C. (1994) 'Parents' views of different respite services', *Mental Handicap Research*, 7(2) 97–117.

Taanila, A., Syrjala, L., Kokkonen, J. and Jarvelin, M. (2002) 'Coping of parents with physically and/or intellectually disabled children', *Child: Care, Health and Development*, 28(1) 73–86.

Teague, B., Fleming, J., Castle, A., Kiernan, B., Lobo, M., Riggs, S. and Wolfe, J. (1993) '"High-tech" home care for children with chronic health conditions: A pilot study', *Journal of Pediatric Nursing*, 8(4) 226–232.

Treneman, M., Corkery, A., Dowdney, L. and Hammond J. (1997) 'Respite-care needs – met and unmet: assessment of needs for children with disability', *Developmental Medicine and Child Neurology*, 39, 548–553.

Valkenier, B., Hayes, V., and McElheran, P. (2002) 'Mothers' perspective of an in-home nursing respite service: coping and control', *Canadian Journal of Nursing Research*, 34(1) 87–109.

While, A., Citrone, C. and Cornish, J. (1996) *A study of the needs and provisions for families caring for children with life-limiting incurable disorders*, London: King's College.

14 Transition to adulthood

Claire Thurgate

The transition from adolescence to adulthood is a challenge for any young person. For those with a disability, and their families, this challenge can be extremely daunting. Some families liken it to 'disappearing into a void' (Morris 2003) as they move from the relative known into the unknown. Consequently, this chapter will aim to explore the statutory process of transition; what tends to occur in reality during transition and what needs to be done to ensure that Transition Planning meets the needs of the young people it is intended to help.

Exploring the statutory process of transition

The legal framework governing the transition process is governed by The Disabled Persons Act (1986), which stipulates the right of the young person to a future needs assessment at the age of fourteen. The Disabled Person Act (1986) is further reinforced by the Code of Practice on the Identification and Assessment of Special Educational Needs (DfEE 1994), which contains a section on transition, advising how the assessment of future need should be undertaken. The initiation of the transition process should include a transitional review meeting (see Appendix 1 of this chapter) for all children over the age of fourteen who have a statement of special education needs. This review should be held at the child's school and involve all those who support the child. The aim of the review is to produce a 'coherent, effective transition plan to support the young person in the last years of school into further education or vocational training' (DfEE 1997). Following on from the transitional review meeting each young person should have a transition plan (see Table 14.1) which identifies six key areas – careers/vocational, academic, health, independence (self-help skills), family/living arrangements and disability benefits/services. Each area needs to be agreed by the young person, parent/carer, school and other agencies. The code of practice on the identification and assessment of special educational needs (DfEE 1994) also includes an overview of the age of transfer from child to adult services (Appendix 2 of this chapter) for young people moving between the different agencies.

Table 14.1 The Transition Plan

Agreed actions by young person, parent/carer, school and other agencies:

Planned Action

CAREERS/VOCATIONAL
Vocational guidance presented in wider context of further education and training courses and should take fully into account the wishes and feelings of the young person.
Work experience arrangements agreed.

ACADEMIC
What are student's curriculum needs during transition?
Is there a plan for integration into another school/college?

HEALTH
Actions required for some young people but not required by the majority.
Role of therapists, special equipment, to be specified.

INDEPENDENCE (Self-help skills)
Consider the degree of support that the young person is likely to need in his/her transition to adult life.

FAMILY/LIVING ARRANGEMENTS
Details of family living arrangements to be achieved.
Action to be taken by agencies involved.

DISABILITY BENEFITS/SERVICES
State the benefits and services currently received.

The Reality of Transition

Transitional review meeting

For some families having the transitional review meeting when the child is aged fourteen may be too early as nineteen, and adulthood, seems a long way away. Consequently, they may not appreciate the importance of such a meeting. Unfortunately, some families are unable to recollect these meetings, or they haven't occurred at all. This may be especially true for young disabled people who are in mainstream schools. If the young person is planning to leave school at sixteen however, a review meeting at fourteen years of age is appropriate. A further difficulty is created by the constant changes that occur within the organisational structures of health, education and social services, which is confusing not only for the young person and their family but also for professionals. Further problems for joint working and information sharing amongst professionals occurs as a result of the different agency boundaries.

The transition plan

This process of planning a young person's future should have them at the centre of it, but frequently the young person doesn't attend the review, or if they do attend, it may be that the professionals talk over their head (Morris 2003). This planning process must ensure that the young person has the information required, in an appropriate format so that they are able to make informed choices. Unfortunately, it appears that this is not always the case and a lack of information is a key barrier identified by young disabled people (ibid.). Parents also require appropriate information so that they are aware of the choices available to their child, but again parents find it difficult to get this information, and have to search for it (ibid.).

Careers/vocational – unfortunately, the careers officer does not always attend the transitional review so the young person is not informed of the opportunities or training courses that may be available, though it may be that there are limited choices and little scope to be creative. On the other hand, some young people may not be able to make informed choices as they are not aware of all the services that are available. Or, because of high levels of need for support young people may be denied access to further education (Angele *et al.* 1996, cited in Morris 2003). If young people with high levels of support needs do continue in further education, it may be at specialist residential colleges, which do not always focus on the development of knowledge, ability and skills. Some 'independent living skills' courses have also been criticised as they focus more on the young people physically doing things for themselves rather than encouraging 'independence of mind' (ibid.) and the ability to live outside a residential environment. Whatever form of career or vocational training the young person undertakes it is imperative that they receive adequate support which must include emotional and developmental support as well as an environment which is supportive of the young person's physical needs.

Academic – the three years prior to the young person leaving school offer a valuable opportunity to deliver specialist training and to prepare for the cultural shift from school to adult life. Unfortunately, for many young people there is often little change between the ages 16–19 from the previous curriculum. Young people need 'real' experiences of post-school options so that they can make informed choices e.g. college or jobs, but in reality many do not have the chance to experience this.

Health – it is imperative that as young people make the transition into adulthood they receive appropriate information about, and access to, healthcare. Unfortunately, many of the services are unfocused and fragmented which will have long-term implications for the young people, with many being prevented from achieving their potential (Chamberlain 1993). Some young people with health needs have been known to their local children's ward for a number of years and may even consider the staff 'part of the family', although in adult services a variety of wards will mean a variety of different staff. Paediatric wards have open visiting hours and parents can stay overnight, while on adult wards there are set visiting times and parents may not be allowed to stay. Within the community the young person will most likely have a community nursing team whom they can contact with any concerns. Once they move to adult services the district nurse may not be easily accessible and the young adult will be expected to use the general practitioner with whom they may have had very little contact in the past. The need for joint clinics to smooth the transition process has been argued for (Chamberlain 1993), but unfortunately the initiation of these clinics remains patchy, although they are appreciated by young people (Pownceby, undated, cited in Morris 2003).

Independent living skills – although the transition plan may specify the degree of support during and following transition, funding issues or lack of service provision may prevent this goal being achieved. Consequently, young people are often not prepared for the major transition into adult life with meetings often focusing on short-term plans and not on longer-term needs. The situation can be further exacerbated if no care manager is appointed.

Family and living arrangements – transition to adulthood is a time when most young people are looking to change their current living arrangements and branch out on their own. This concept of independence is difficult for most young people, but young disabled people face even more barriers – they are less likely to be employed and the private rent section has less to offer in terms of specially adapted housing. This situation can be compounded by the fact that representatives from Housing rarely attend the transitional review meeting. The young person requires appropriate information about choices for accommodation, but it appears that this doesn't always happen, nor is the young person always involved in the decision-making process (Morris 2003). As part of their package of care many young people may be accessing respite services, which they may want to continue into adulthood. However, it appears that there can be a lack of availability and choice of adult respite services. Consequently, as a result of a lack of respite and other forms of independent living arrangements it is presumed that the young person will live at home or move to residential care (Morris 2003). Both of these options may be fraught with difficulties – parents will be getting older and may not be physically able to care for their child and many residential homes do not cater for young adults.

Disability benefits and services – families will have become familiar with the benefits and services available to their child and become shocked by the changes, which occur once the young person leaves school. Unfortunately, many young people and their families are not informed of the changes within the benefit system. Nor are adult services informed early enough about each individual young person's needs. Many young people will reach adulthood with no appropriate services in place. Sadly, for some young people social and leisure activities can be extremely limited and this is likely to be further limited for those young people who have more significant impairments (Hirst and Baldwin 1994). By denying young people the opportunity to socialise their 'personal and social development' suffers as a result (Morris 2003). For others, services may be available, but young people are prevented from accessing them as there are transport issues. It may be that transport is no longer funded, or there is limited equipment available to aid their mobility.

Implications for practice

1 The young person needs to be involved in the planning of the transition process to ensure that the outcomes are user led and not service led. For this situation to occur it is imperative that inclusive consultation and planning begins early. This will ensure the information required by the young person, to make choices, is available. No matter how severe the young person's impairment they will be able to contribute in a meaningful way if they receive appropriate assistance. One way that this may be achieved is through the use of talking mats (Cameron and Murphy 2002). Talking mats is a pictorial framework that uses three sets of picture symbols – topics that are relevant to transition, options which relate to each topic and emotions that allow the young person to indicate their general feeling about each option. Each mat focuses on one topic – there are six topics in all, so that the young person is not overloaded with information. The use of person-centred plans is another way in which young people may be able to communicate their wishes and aspirations for the future, as well as those things they don't like. The young person may choose who they would like to help them with their 'plan', but what is important is that the young person is at the centre of the plan. The person-centred plan should address what the young person likes now, what they don't like and what their strengths are. The young person will also have the opportunity to indicate what is important to them i.e. living on their own, what is required to achieve this and who will be involved. The use of communication passports may also be of use during the transition process as these contain a great deal of personal information about the young person.
2 Communication support is imperative for the young person and their family during the transition period. Not only will it aid the use of talking mats, person-centred plans and communication; it also ensures that the young person has the information, in a format that they understand, to make informed choices. To overcome communication difficulties it may be necessary to use a creative approach. Two ways of informing the young person of the choices available are through personal experience or the use of audio-visual equipment. The use of an advocate or facilitator who works in speech and language therapy will ensure that the information provided is not too complex, as well as supporting the student's contribution. When meetings are planned it is important to support the young person ensuring that they are relaxed and the environment is

familiar. This will prevent them from becoming overwhelmed by the situation.

3 Information is required by the young person, and their family, so that they are able to make informed choices. This information should be given in the most appropriate form for the individual to understand, and written information must also be given to the family.

4 Work by Pownceby (undated, cited in Morris 2003), during the transition period, found that young people with cystic fibrosis wanted support from paediatric staff and welcome from adult staff; to see the paediatrician alone for sometime before transition; transferring as part of a group; practical written information about the new centre; joint clinics; a chance to visit new centre; a longer period of preparation and the chance to talk about anxieties. Young people need to be prepared for in-patient stays as well as out-patient clinics, especially as many of these young people will have had open access to their paediatric wards or would have spent considerable amounts of time on the unit. One area that could be looked at would be to introduce the young person to the adult wards and their protocols or have young people wards, from 18–25 years, so that young adults are not on wards with older patients. Viner (1999) has a number of recommendations for best practice for transition (see Appendix 3 of this chapter). One of his recommendations is for a specific transition policy. This is imperative, for in the United Kingdom no single model of transition has been adopted as standard (Soanes *et al.* 2004).

5 It appears that many general practitioners are poorly equipped, for whatever reason, to coordinate transition care. Therefore, general practitioners need to be more closely involved with the young persons' care leading up to transition.

6 To ensure that the transition to adult services is a positive and purposeful process with the young person at the centre, the planning must involve partnership and joint working with the many professionals involved. An identified transition worker for health, social services and education would aid this process.

7 The Royal College of Nursing Adolescent Health Forum (2004) has published 'Adolescent transition care: guidance for nursing staff' which recognises that transition must be a guided, educational therapeutic process rather than an administration event. The transition guidance (RCN 2004) includes a very useful sample of a planning checklist, and evidence record, which can be facilitated using a competency-based framework. The framework covers six key areas:

- Self-advocacy.
- Independent healthcare behaviour.
- Sexual health.
- Psychosocial support.

- Educational and vocational planning.
- Health and lifestyle.

at each of the three stages of transition: early, middle and late. This framework can be used in conjunction with the RCN's (2004) own clinical pathway which if used generically could promote consistent standards and processes throughout the health service. It is hoped that the full National Service Framework will cover transition in its broadest sense to include social care, education and employment, so that the process can be more than just lip service.

References

Royal College of Nursing (2004) *Adolescent transition care: guidance for nursing staff*, London: Adolescent Health Forum.

Cameron, L. and Murphy, J. (2002) 'Enabling young people with a learning disability to make choices at a time of transition', *British Journal of Learning Disabilities*, 30, 105–112.

Chamberlain, M. A. (1993) 'Physically handicapped school leavers?', *Archives of Disease in Childhood*, 69, 399–402.

Department of Health (1986) *The Disabled Person Act*, London: HMSO.

Department for Early Education (1994) *The Identification and Assessment of Special Educational Needs*, London: HMSO.

Department for Early Education (1997) *Primary and Secondary Education in England and Wales: From 1944*, London: HMSO.

Hirst, M. and Baldwin, S. (1994) *Unequal opportunities: growing up disabled*. London: HMSO.

Morris, J. (2003) *Hurtling into a void: transition to adulthood for young disabled people with 'complex health and support needs'*, London: Pavilion.

Soanes, C. and Timmons, S. (2004) 'Improving transition: a qualitative study examining the attitudes of young people with chronic illness transferring to adult care', *Journal of Child Health Care*, 8 (2) 103–112.

Viner, R. (1999) 'Transition from paediatric to adult care: Bridging the gaps or passing the buck?', *Archives of Disease in Childhood*, 81, 271–275.

APPENDIX 1

The Transition Review Meeting (Code of practice on the identification and assessment of special educational needs, DfEE 1994).

LEAD AGENCY:

Education

WHO IS IT FOR?

All young people over 14 years with a Statement of Special Educational Needs

WHO ATTENDS?

School: Head Teacher, Special Educational Needs Co-ordinator, Integrated Support Service, Class Teacher, Classroom Assistant (variable)
Local Education Authority Representative
Careers/Vocational Guidance
Educational Psychologist (if involved)
Social Services: Social Worker (if involved)
Health: School Medical Officer, Therapies (if involved)
Transitional Worker (if available)
Parent-Carers
Young Person

WHERE?

At the school

TIME SCALE:

Notice given two months before Transitional Review Meeting (but not a requirement); information circulated two weeks prior to meeting; report prepared and circulated one week after Transitional Review Meeting.

WHAT IS THE STATED PURPOSE OF THE TRANSITIONAL REVIEW MEETING?

'To review the statement of special education needs to agree objectives and targets and ultimately produce a coherent, effective transition plan to support the young person in the last years of school into further education or vocational training.' (Transition planning: Transition from the age of 14 years to adulthood. DfEE 1997).

APPENDIX 2

Age of transfer from children to adult services

AGENCY	AGE
Social Services	18 years
Education	16–19 years
Health	16 or 19 years
Careers	14 years
Transitional Support Worker	14–20 years
Case Worker	N/A

APPENDIX 3

Recommendations for best practice (Viner 1999)

- Transition preparation must be seen as an essential component of high quality health care in adolescence.

- Every paediatric general and speciality clinic should have a specific transition policy. More formal transition programmes are necessary where large numbers of young people are being transferred to adult care.

- Young people should not be transferred to adult services until they have the necessary skills to function in an adult service and have finished growth and puberty.

- An identified person within the paediatric and adult teams must be responsible for transition arrangements. The most suitable persons are nurse specialists.

- Management links must be developed between the two hospitals. Within the new NHS, contracting and financing issues must be worked out in detail. Local commissioners must be consulted when patients are transferred from one tertiary centre to another.

- Large children services should develop a 'transition map' detailing where and how transfer occurs speciality by speciality.

- Evaluation of transition arrangements must be undertaken.

15 The way forward

Helen K. Warner

It should be clear by now that good practice when caring for children with disabilities in the acute setting requires close collaboration both with the families themselves, and with all other professionals, from health, education and social services, who are involved with the child and family. The difficulties experienced by nurses when attempting to do this may be reflected in the difficulties experienced by the child/young person themselves. It seems that every aspect of life that most of us take for granted is not only more difficult but often dependent on the help of others. If we consider the difficulties many of us so-called able-bodied people have, in asking for help with every-day matters, then it becomes possible to begin to understand the painful reality that is often the lives of those with a disability and especially those with a learning disability.

Models of practice

Recognising that no one discipline, in isolation, can meet the needs of these children enables us to understand that no one model or theory should be relied on in practice to meet the childrens's needs. Kelly (2004) suggests that while models of practice enable practitioners to work within healthcare systems so that they become competent, they may also inhibit continuing professional development towards expert practice. Kelly argues that, although competent practitioners may be able to use a model of practice and apply it in different situations, the expert practitioner is able to act outside the constraints of particular models or situations and suit his/her actions to the needs that his/her experience and expertise identify. Thus a few concepts from a variety of theories may be selected and used to develop a personal model of practice (Reed and Sanderson 1999). Reed and Sanderson (1999) and Kelly (2004) were discussing occupational therapy practice but their arguments could equally apply to children's nursing.

In order to meet the children's needs holistically, we need to begin to think in a more holistic way, and this means broadening our knowledge base so that even if we may not be expert in other areas of knowledge, we can confidently use that knowledge to inform our work, and at the very least recognise our own limitations more clearly, and know when to refer on to a more appropriate colleague or service. Models of practice are intended to guide clinical reasoning but not to dictate it (Kelly 2004) and if we believe in the uniqueness of individual children the use of one model is precluded. Although nursing theory is obviously important and a good foundation, it is also important to recognise that the theories used by other health professionals all overlap, so that we also need to draw from theories such as sensory integration theory, psychodynamic and psychoanalytical theories, transactional analysis and social judgement theory, and the theories and models used by occupational therapists, physiotherapists, speech and language therapists and psychologists, as well as medical colleagues. Above all it is important to understand that the medical model itself has elements of conveying powerlessness (Burke 2004), while the social model of disability can be empowering. Thus a combination of models and a multi-disciplinary approach with multi-disciplinary assessments has to be the way forward. Multi-agency assessments will need to be considered when discharge planning is undertaken to ensure that the child and family have the appropriate support, and that all agencies involved are aware of the latest developments.

Unfortunately the National Health Service is structured so that traditionally there has been a splitting of the psychological needs of children from the medical needs which seems ludicrous when one considers the powerful effects that the mind has on the body and which is shown so clearly in sensory integration theory and psychodynamic and psychoanalytical theories. Thankfully this situation is beginning to be addressed as awareness is raised that the mental health needs of children and young people are every nurse's business (RCN 2004). However much remains to be done and there are implications for further training and awareness of these issues, particularly when it comes to children with learning disabilities and challenging behaviour. Successful interventions for these children depend on staff having a broad knowledge base in relation to safe reactive strategies, psychological and behavioural approaches and long-term skills teaching strategies (DoH 1993). However, (McKenzie *et al.* 2004) have shown that the beliefs people have about the cause of the behaviour, affect how they respond to it, and the need for appropriate training is highlighted.

Joint training

Reeves and Freeth (2000) demonstrated that the provision of joint training for medical, nursing, physiotherapy and occupational therapy students enables them to develop appropriate attitudes as well as knowledge and skills. Once qualified, the students are then more able to work collaboratively. Working together in this way can only serve to improve communication and understanding between professions and ultimately a reduction in individual frustrations (Freeman 1999). However, although individual practitioners may be willing to change their practice the framework and support also need to be in place to make this happen. The National Framework for children, and the Children's Bill, which became the Children Act 2004, and which has come from the government paper Every Child Matters (2003), are intended to address this by focusing on early intervention, preventative work and integrated services for children through children's trusts. Alongside these proposed changes, the government's strategy, 'Removing Barriers to Achievement' (DfES 2004) sets out a programme of sustained action and review, both nationally and locally, for the education of children with special educational needs. Thus all services are changing and moving forward together towards more integrated ways of working so that the opportunities for children to reach their potential will be ensured. However, we are not there yet, although this is an exciting time of change and opportunity for professionals as well as for children and families.

Complex needs

According to the Council for Disabled Children (2002) children with autism and children dependent on complex medical technology continue to increase in numbers and have been identified by local authorities as being the greatest challenge to services. These children have complex needs. However, the term 'complex health and support needs' that tends to be used by professionals and policy makers can be confusing. It is the systems and services that have to be negotiated in order to access a good quality of life that are complex, and existing services seemingly find it complex to meet the needs of children, asserts Morris (1999). Arguments about who should provide a service or piece of equipment continue, and remain central to decisions about service provision; in addition, changing definitions of health and social care add to the confusion (Leneham *et al.* 2004). Despite the report by a Select Committee of the House of Commons on children's health in the community (1997), there is still a lack of advice and direction for local services to reach joint agreements.

Mencap (2001) describes children with learning disabilities and health needs being excluded from education, in spite of policy guidance to reasonably manage the risks (Servian *et al.* 1998). Confusion and uncertainty remain about who is responsible for children's healthcare needs at school. Leneham *et al.* (2004) argue that joint risk management is needed, which should be supported by joint protocols and funding, and suggest that Children's Trusts may be able to meet this need.

Children's Trusts

Children's Trusts have arisen from the government's green paper, 'Every Child Matters' (2003), as the preferred way forward to achieve the five main outcomes for children identified in the paper as: being healthy, staying safe, enjoying and achieving, making a positive contribution and economic well-being. The director of Children's Services will have responsibility for all the Trusts' services, and for coordinating services outside of the organisation.

Children's Trusts are intended to integrate key local services – education, social care and health services for children and young people. They incorporate integrated commissioning strategies delivered through a range of providers that are designed to meet local evaluations of need. Trusts may also include other services i.e. Connexions (a youth service that provides advice, guidance and personal development services for 13–19 year olds); Youth Offending Teams; Sure Start, and other local partners i.e. the police, voluntary organisations, housing and leisure services. Most areas should have a Children's Trust by 2006, and Primary Care Trusts will be able to pool funds with local authorities. This should lead to improved and joined up services, which can respond to the needs of children and families rather than children and families having to adapt to the needs of services. As a consequence of this, there should be less frustration for the children and families themselves and also for the people who deliver the services. Further information about Children's Trusts can be found at: www.dfes.gov.uk/childrenstrusts/. There is currently a three-year national evaluation study in progress, of the 35 pathfinder Trusts, which is intended to build up an evidence base to contribute to the development of practice and policy for future Children's Trusts.

The development of Children's Trusts is a positive way to integrate services at a strategic level. However, legislation alone is not enough, as we have seen before e.g. with the Disability Discrimination Act (1995), and attitudes and beliefs are much more difficult to change.

Valuing people and their skills

Perhaps of equal importance to an integrated framework is for senior managers to recognise and value people with disabilities and the staff who work with them. Respect for this client group should be reflected in respect for the staff and this needs to be demonstrated, by providing staff with opportunities for training and education to develop the skills they need to be able to adequately care for these children. Often the needs for further training and development take second place to training opportunities for acute care and this will have an impact on the care provided. Similarly, care staff in residential settings are frequently devalued, attributed little respect and deemed not worthy of training (Mattison and Pistrang 2004) and yet they are expected to implement complicated and demanding work to manage and support clients with complex needs.

However, the skills required to care for children with disabilities are skills that will enhance the care of all children. It is no longer acceptable to assume that nurses, and indeed any professional, can communicate well without additional training. No doubt we can all think of clinicians who may have excellent knowledge of their area of expertise but whose communication with children, families and colleagues, leaves a great deal to be desired. Good communication is a skill to be learnt, like any other, and should not be left to chance, particularly as it will also affect the individual's ability to manage stress, and nursing is acknowledged as an occupation with one of the highest levels of stress (Roger and Nash 1993; Seymour 1995). Chatterton (1999) showed that a combination of direct speech and language therapy input and communication training, effectively improved communication between nurses and people with learning disabilities. It was suggested by the Royal College of Speech and Language Therapists (1996) that the focus of training should be on developing the understanding of staff and carers of the role of the environment and the effect that their own communication has on the behaviour of the individual with a learning disability. Above all it is vital to be sensitive to feedback from the child, respecting their cues.

Support

Good support is another vital component, and a great deal has been written about the need to feel cared for to be able to care for others. Clinical supervision is therefore not a luxury, but essential if children's nurses and other health professionals are to feel adequately supported and able to remain focused on the needs of the client group. There has also been a great deal written about good support of staff reducing sick levels and burnout. Since the NHS's workforce is its greatest resource, valuing the people who work in it and their people skills is long overdue. There are often drives to recruit staff into the caring professions, but far less attention is paid to retaining existing and experienced staff. Surely it must be more cost effective, having trained and educated health professionals over several years, to ensure their working conditions meet their needs. Nurses have a duty of care to provide good quality care to their clients (NMC 2002). However, in order to do so, they must have the resources to do so and this includes having their own needs met by the provision of appropriate support.

Early intervention

We also know that early intervention works, and this is recognised in *Every Child Matters* (DoH 2003), and yet there is a national shortage not only of children's nurses but also of occupational therapists, physiotherapists, speech and language therapists, clinical psychologists, counsellors and social workers, so that so many of these children, and their families, are unable to access the support they require at an early stage, in order to prevent further problems and family breakdown at a later stage (Utting 1995). Current services can only offer the barest minimum support and sometimes not even that. In the long term this can only lead to ingrained problems which are more difficult to deal with and the associated costs both in human and social terms as well as financial.

In a study of children with Usher Syndrome, Sherlock (2000, cited in Shampan 2002) found that 78 per cent of participants would have welcomed counselling services but did not get it due to not knowing where to go, or because of long waiting lists. One can only guess at the distress caused for parents who need immediate emotional help being placed on a waiting list. It is also important to remember that it is not only the individual's inner struggle for acceptance that is so painful but also the lack of sufficient acceptance in society that is an ongoing source of distress for families.

Creative thinking

Ideally there would be more children's trained nurses to reflect the needs of these children, and a paediatric occupational therapist attached to each paediatric ward to advise on positioning and equipment. Thinking creatively and outside of the box can lead to simple but effective solutions. Rotational posts between children's wards and special care baby units; children's wards and child development centres; and learning disability community services and acute children's services are not beyond the realms of possibility. Neither are visits to special schools, and closer links with school nurses, impossible to consider. These would all improve communication and understanding of disability issues, while also broadening the knowledge base of nurses, not to mention increased job satisfaction.

These suggestions may be idealistic for an overworked and under-resourced NHS, but there needs to be an acknowledgement, at organisational level, that quality practice requires time and resources (Warner 2001), and this includes adequate numbers of staff. However, commitment to a shared set of principles and a positive attitude can motivate people to work together in multi-disciplinary/multi-agency teams as the writer is able to acknowledge from personal experience. Managing the care of children with disabilities and their families is an art as well as a science. With the current focus so heavily on technological advancements it is easy to lose sight of the art of nursing and yet this aspect of human caring is of equal importance if we are to truly respect the children and families as fellow human beings, and it is the very essence of nursing. Studying art and literature can make a vital contribution to nurses' different 'ways of knowing,' asserts Darbyshire (1994) in his description of a course entitled, 'Understanding caring through arts and humanities'. If we are to restore the balance between the art and science of nursing then nurse education perhaps needs to follow this lead and give more attention to the art of nursing.

Quality care

Disabled children should have the right to the same quality of care that all children have (Leneham *et al.* 2004). A proactive approach needs to be taken to risk management and ultimately to the inclusion of disabled children into everyday life. It is mainstream services that need to change and develop to embrace diversity, and this means recognising that all children can communicate and have something valuable to say, and finding ways to enable them to do so (ibid.). This means providing services to meet children's needs and not expecting children to fit into services. Understanding individual communication helps everyone relate to the child and be able to read the early signs of happiness and distress. The creative use of communication passports is a way of ensuring that everyone involved with the child has the same information and can provide a consistent approach. Not only do they tell us how the person communicates and how to interpret it, but also how to give them information in a way they can understand. We must also remember that children have a legal right to be included in decisions about matters that affect them (DOH 1991) and that we may empower them to be included by listening to their views (Lovett 1996; Burke 2004). As we saw in Chapter 4, if society can be judged by the actions it takes, a caring and civilized society means that we must take good care of our most vulnerable members.

Quality care is also about understanding the impact of caring on families, which spans the physical, psychological and social domains (Cairns 1992; Barr 1997), so that effective interventions must also do the same. It is essential that we do not make assumptions, and remember that while there may be pain, suffering and sorrow, there may also be joy, hope and optimism (Kearney and Griffin 2001). Burke (2004) reminds us that the impact of caring for a disabled child will also have an effect on the disabled child's siblings, a population whose needs are still often overlooked even though they may be taking on some of the tasks of caring on a daily basis. For this reason, siblings too need to be included in discussions with the family about current and future events regarding the disabled child or they may lose confidence and suffer a lowered self-esteem (Dyson 1996). As suggested in Chapter 10, a family system's approach is required; this may also include grandparents as they attempt to support their own child as well as their grandchild.

Quality care is working in partnership with children, their families and the other professionals who support them. It means including children in quality measures and audit and ensuring that their 'voice' is heard and understood (Moules 2004). Information on materials available for working with disabled children can be found at (www.doh./integratedchildrenssystem). The Children's Society (1999; 2002) and the NSPCC/TRIANGLE /JRF (2001) have also produced materials to enhance communication with disabled children. However, for children's nurses this is an area that is deserving of more attention and further training.

Quality care means having good links with community services so that there is continuity of care when these children are discharged from the acute setting and also during the transition into adult services as children move into adolescence and adulthood. This involves planning in advance to ensure that potential obstacles can be anticipated and removed as far as possible. Above all it means adequate preparation.

Preparation, preparation, preparation

The importance of preparation for these children cannot be over-emphasised. Prevention is better than cure and in keeping with the ethos of this book it is important to consider the kind of preparation that may be undertaken prior to a child's admission. Changing a child's routine can cause them anxiety especially if their understanding is limited in any way. Children can be supported to manage changes if the adults around them take time to prepare them in a way the child can understand.

There must be an acknowledgement by nurses that parents will need to communicate to their child what will happen and when (Aylott 2000). Inviting parents to the ward before the admission will enable them to understand the admission process themselves so that they can feel confident when preparing their child. Photographs of the hospital and ward entrances, the ward environment and if possible of one or two members of staff who will be on duty when the child is to be admitted can go some way towards reducing the child's anxiety, in addition to allowing them to bring along something from home that makes them feel safe e.g. a favourite toy or comforter.

It will also be important to be aware that the child may be hyper-sensitive to sensory input i.e. lighting, noise e.g. from ward televisions, or smell or even all three of these, and to ask his/her parents what will help to make them comfortable during the admission.

Another way of preparing a child for hospital appointments or admissions is by the creation of a social story. The concept of the social story was developed by Carol Gray, for children with autism. Examples of social stories can be found in Gray and White (2002) on the following websites: (www.autism.org/stories.html; www.thegraycentre.org). These are literal/concrete stories written in the first person and which deal with the who, what, when and why of experience. The story is customised to suit the child's particular needs and works at a conscious level with the child's cognition, to aid their understanding by describing, instructing, informing and reassuring. Literal accuracy is ensured by use of the words, 'sometimes' and 'usually' and the title should be brief and state the story's meaning e.g. 'a story about going to hospital'.

Therapeutic stories (Sunderland 2000), on the other hand, help children think about and process difficult emotions. The child's difficult emotions and circumstances are translated into metaphor and symbolism through the story. The everyday language of feeling ('I'm sad') is inadequate and does not describe the richness of experience in the same way as a story. Using metaphor enables the child to think about difficult feelings from a safe distance, and it is important *not* to come out of metaphor unless the child does. The story highlights how the child's current behaviour/coping mechanisms are maladaptive and should show the main character using more appropriate strategies and resolving the situation. Therapeutic stories work on the imagination at an unconscious level, and need to be read to the child repeatedly. You know they are being effective and the message getting through, if the child actively seeks out the story and requests for it to be read to them.

Obviously the ways of preparing children for admission described above need time to implement and will not be appropriate in an emergency situation. However, they could be considered for all routine admissions. Once the initial work is undertaken, it is not too difficult to replicate and customise for individual children. Yes, resources like time and paper will be needed, but children's experiences of hospital can be enhanced, the fear and mystery removed, and challenging behaviours that may require more costly resources, such as extra staff, can be avoided.

From the above, and previous chapters, it is clear that a great deal can be done, by individual practitioners to improve the quality of the hospital experience for children with disabilities. This is not enough in itself, and changes need to be made at organisational and strategic levels to ensure that these vulnerable children are no longer denied what they have a right to expect according to the United Nations Convention on the Rights of the Child (1989). Joint funding and working between health, education and social services has to be the way forward to meet the needs of children with disabilities and their families. More work also needs to be done from the child or young person's own perspective in order for their views to be heard.

When services are finally able to meet the needs of children with disabilities and their families consistently, and adapt to the families' changing requirements, children's nursing will have taken a giant step forward, for we will have learnt how to work collaboratively with colleague health professionals as well as with colleagues from other agencies. We will also have learnt to balance the art and science of nursing and to value them both equally. Perhaps most importantly of all we will have learnt how to work in true partnership with the children and families themselves. This will provide a model of collaborative care from which all children could benefit and indeed, adult services too.

References

Aylott, J. (2000) 'Understanding children with autism: exploding the myths', *British Journal of Nursing*, 9(12) 779–784.

Barr, O. (1997) 'Interventions in a family context', chapter 16 in B. Gates (ed.) *Learning Disabilities* (3rd edn) London: Churchill Livingstone.

Burke, P. (2004) *Brothers and Sisters of Disabled Children*, London: Jessica Kingsley.

Cairns, I. (1992) 'The health of mothers and fathers with a child with a disability', *Health Visitor*, 65, 238–239.

Chatterton, S. (1999) 'Communication skills workshops in learning disability nursing', *British Journal of Nursing*, 8(2) 90–96.

Children's Society (1999) *I'll Go First: The planning and review Kit for use with Children with disabilities*, London: Children's Society.

Children's Society (2002) *Ask Us* (CD-Rom), Commissioned by the Quality Protects Reference Group.

Council for Disabled Children (2002) *Fourth Analysis of the Quality Protects Management Action Plans: Services for disabled children and their families*, London: CDC.

Darbyshire, P. (1994) 'Understanding caring through arts and humanities: a medical/nursing humanities approach to promoting alternative experiences of thinking and learning', *Journal of Advanced Nursing*, 19, 856–863.

Department of Education and Skills (2004) *Removing Barriers to Achievement*, London: DfES.

Department of Health (1991) *The Children Act 1989: Guidance & Regulations: Vol. 6 Children with Disabilities: A New Framework for the Care & Upbringing of Children*, London: HMSO.

Department of Health (1995) *Disability Discrimination Act*, London: HMSO.

Department of Health (2003) *Every Child Matters*, London: HMSO.

Department of Health (2004) *The Children Act*, London: HMSO.

Dyson, L. (1996) 'The experience of families of children with learning disabilities: Parental stress, family functioning and sibling self-concept', *Journal of Learning Disabilities*, 2(9) 280–286.

Freeman, M. (1999) 'Can different healthcare professionals really work as a team?' *Nursing Management*, 6(7) 10–13.

Gray, C. and White, A. L. (2002) *My Social Stories Book*, London: Jessica Kingsley.

HMSO (1997) *Health Services for Children and Young People in the Community, Home and School*, Third Report.

Kearney, P. M. and Griffin, T. (2001) 'Between joy and sorrow: being a parent of a child with developmental disability', *Journal of Advanced Nursing*, 34(5) 582–592.

Kelly, G. (2004) 'Paediatric Occupational Therapy in the 21st Century: A Survey of UK Practice', *NAPOT Journal* (National Association of Paediatric Occupational Therapists), Summer, 8(2) 5–8.

Lenehan, C., Morrison, J. and Stanley, J. (2004) *The Dignity of Risk: a practical handbook for professionals working with disabled children and their families*, London: Council for Disabled Children; Shared Care Network.

Lovett, H. (1996) *Learning to Listen: Positive Approaches and People with Difficult Behaviour*, Baltimore: Paul Brookes.

Mattison, V. and Pistrang, N. (2004) 'The endings of relationships between people with learning disabilities and their Keyworkers', chapter 11 in D. Simpson and L. Miller (eds) *Unexpected Gains: Psychotherapy with People with Learning Disabilities*, London: Karnac Books.

McKenzie, K., Paxton, D., Loads, D., Kwaitek, E., McGregor, L. and Sharp, K. (2004) 'The impact of nurse education on staff attributions in relation to challenging behaviour', *Learning Disability Practice* 7 (5) June, 16–20.

Mencap (2001) *Don't Count me Out: The exclusion of children with a learning disability from education because of health needs*, London: Mencap.

Morris, J. (1999) *Hurtling into the Void*, London: Pavilion.

Moules, T. (2004) 'Whose Quality is it? Young people report on a participatory research project to explore the involvement of children in monitoring quality of care in hospital', *Paediatric Nursing*, 16(6) August, 30–31.

NSPCC/TRIANGLE/JRF (2001) *Two Way Street*, a training video and handbook about communicating with disabled children and young people.

Nursing Midwifery Council (2002) *Code of Professional Conduct*, NMC.

Reed, K. L. and Sanderson, S. N. (1999) *Concepts of Occupational Therapy*, Philadelphia: Lippincott, Williams and Wilkins.

Reeves, S. and Freeth, D. (2000) Learning to Collaborate, *Nursing Times*, 13(96) 40–41.

Roger, D. and Nash, P. (1993) 'Smart Delivery', *Nursing Times*, July 14, 89(28) 30–31.

Royal College Nursing (2004) *Children and Young People's Mental Health: Every Nurse's Business*, London: RCN.

Royal College of Speech & Language Therapists (1996) *Communicating Quality 2*, London: Royal College of Speech & Language Therapists.

Salvage, J. (2000) 'Working with dinasours', *Nursing Times*, 96(13) 23.

Servian, R., Jones, V., Lenehan, C. and Spires, S. (1998) *Towards a Healthy Future: Multi-agency working in the management of invasive and life-saving procedures for children in family based services*, Bristol: The Policy Press.

Seymour, J. (1995) 'Counting the Cost', *Nursing Times*, May 31 (91) 22, 24–27.

Shampan, L. (2002) *Parents have Needs too! The role of counselling services for children with special needs and disabilities*, 3C's Counselling Service (Community Counselling for Carers of Children with Special Needs), Ealing: Mencap.

Sunderland, M. (2000) *Using Story Telling as a Therapeutic Tool with children*, London: Winslow Press.

United Nations (1989) *The Convention on the Rights of the Child*, Geneva: United Nations Children Fund.

Utting, W. (1995) *Family and Parenthood: Supporting Families, Preventing Breakdown*, York: Joseph Rowntree Foundation.

Warner, H. (2001) 'Children with additional needs: The transdisciplinary approach', *Paediatric Nursing*, July 13 (6) 33–3.

Index

Page numbers in *italics* refer to tables; *a* indicates appendix.